T0175470

BEYOND
THE TOOLKIT

BEYOND
THE TOOLKIT
LEADING QUALITY IMPROVEMENT IN HEALTH AND SOCIAL CARE

BRIAN MARSHALL LIZ WIGGINS JANET SMALLWOOD
with contributors

Endorsements for Beyond the Toolkit

Successive attempts, successes and failures in improvement in health and care have taught us that whilst methodology and approach are important, the focus must be less on the intervention and more on the context. This book provides a compelling collection of insights into the work of leadership as intervention, drawn from our flagship GenerationQ leadership programme. Moving "beyond the toolkit" and into the complex, challenging, emotional and human reality that sets the context within which leaders at all levels seek to create the conditions where meaningful improvements in performance can occur. A powerful collection of stories that provide hope and inspiration to us all.

Dr Jennifer Dixon, Chief Executive, The Health Foundation

We are in a time of unprecedented change, and in health care, we urgently need new ways to lead and to improve. This book *Beyond the Toolkit* is an important way to learn more in both domains. Transforming health care at this pace needs new skills at building the will for change, new ideas and models for care, and the methods for executing and spreading these changes to all. The stories in this book demonstrate the leadership attributes needed for will-building and the tools for harvesting great ideas and introducing them reliably across our complex systems. It's a perfect marriage of meaning and methods. It's filled with practical ways to build personal leadership expertise and examples of how to use those skills for the team-building so vital for improving.

Maureen Bisognano, President Emerita,
Institute for Healthcare Improvement

Beyond the Toolkit is a leadership book for real-life leaders of health care services. It explores theory with a light touch giving prominence to the inspiring stories of people leading improvement and how they use the framework presented to reflect and develop their skills through lived experience. How wonderful to share their deep personal insights into their leadership acts, motivations and vulnerabilities. A must-read for all health care leaders.

Dr Joanna Bircher, Clinical Director of GM GP Excellence,
Programme Board member Advancing Quality Alliance

Deeply personal and disarmingly honest, the stories of improvement recounted by GenerationQ Fellows are expertly curated. *Beyond the Toolkit* is anchored in the everyday challenges we all face working in complex health and care systems. Yes the tools are important, but even more valuable to our improvement endeavours are the relationships we nurture, the choices we make and our ability to understand ourselves and our context. Stories from the frontline – all a rich tapestry of learning! The authors have served the GenerationQ programme and our Fellowship very well.

Dr Lourda Geoghegan, Director Quality Improvement & Medical Director
Regulation & Quality Improvement Authority, Belfast

This is the perfect book for those who believe that quality improvement is more than just the "method". It takes the reader on a journey from defining quality improvement through to how to create the culture that QI needs for it to thrive in an organisation. The real-life examples are fantastic at bringing a real-life feel to the text.

Jonathan Warren, Acting Chief Executive,
Surrey and Borders Partnership NHS Foundation Trust

The real-life stories which are unafraid to shine a light on the very real personal challenges faced by leaders resonate with all of us trying to lead in the health and social care system. Any leader or aspiring leader reading this book will recognise situations from which they can draw parallels but also read how a change in approach can provide inspiration and examples of where small gestures can make a big impact for a leader, their teams and patients.

Jatinder Harchowal, Chief Pharmacist / Clinical Director,
Medicines Management & Clinical Support Services,
The Royal Marsden NHS Foundation Trust

A "go-to" resource for NHS and public-sector leaders in tough jobs managing change and service delivery in tough environments. Written through the eyes and experiences of real people working through big issues against the pressure of delivering services that we all rely on.

Richard Lee QAM, Director of Operations,
Welsh Ambulance Services NHS Trust

This book takes a refreshing look at leadership, blending the human element with context and technical aspects. An insightful and powerful foray into leadership and quality improvement through personal stories that could just change how you view yourself and others! A book to keep at hand to help prod that professional curiosity.

Mark Brassington, Chief Operating Officer,
United Lincolnshire Hospitals Trust

As a medical student, I so wished I'd read this before undertaking the mandatory QI project during my fourth year. This book inspired and motivated me far more than my university teaching on the subject as it helped me see more clearly the rationale for QI and the human side.

Ellie Richards, 5th-year medical student,
King's College, University of London

These are real stories of improving quality in the NHS – so much more than idealistic theory, the authors have produced a highly relatable guide to the messiness of leading change in the real world whilst dealing with all the other stuff that life throws at you. An essential read for anyone who is looking to produce sustainable improvements by not only applying the theory but understanding their own impact on their colleagues and patients.

Andy Heeps, Divisional Director, Specialist Medicine,
Barking, Havering and Redbridge University Hospitals NHS Trust

First published in 2018 by Libri Publishing

Copyright © Ashridge (Bonar Law Memorial) Trust

The right of Brian Marshall, Liz Wiggins and Janet Smallwood to be identified as the authors of this work has been asserted in accordance with the Copyright, Designs and Patents Act, 1988.

ISBN: 978-1-911450-17-7

All rights reserved. No part of this publication may be reproduced, stored in any retrieval system or transmitted in any form or by any means, electronic, mechanical, photocopying, recording or otherwise, without the prior written permission of the copyright holder for which application should be addressed in the first instance to the publishers. No liability shall be attached to the author, the copyright holder or the publishers for loss or damage of any nature suffered as a result of reliance on the reproduction of any of the contents of this publication or any errors or omissions in its contents.

A CIP catalogue record for this book is available from The British Library

Cover and book design by Carnegie Publishing
Reprinted in 2019 by Halstan UK

Libri Publishing
Brunel House
Volunteer Way
Faringdon
Oxfordshire
SN7 7YR

Tel: +44 (0)845 873 3837

www.libripublishing.co.uk

Acknowledgements

Writing a book of this sort never involves the effort of the authors alone but particularly because this book is a collection of stories, there are some special thanks to be said. The book represents a great deal of thinking and learning together, involving challenge and support.

Firstly, we would like to thank those senior health leaders who were willing to share their experiences and take the time to write their stories on top of busy clinical, leadership and family commitments. These are Chris Barben, Charles Daniels, George Findlay, Aideen Keaney, Annie Laverty, Paul McArdle, Sarah Marriott, Fiona Pender, Ed Rysdale, Hiro Tanaka, Peter Wilson and Frances Wiseman. Their gesture in sharing their stories represents true courage, real generosity, and a deeply felt desire to help others working in a system that they, and we, care about. Their willingness to put themselves out there by sharing their experiences, with the intention of helping other leaders to improve the quality of care for patients, service users, carers and staff, is something we applaud, appreciate and admire.

Their ability to lead, to be brave, to experiment and to then tell their stories and share their learning has not been a solo endeavour. It has been made possible by the numerous conversations that have taken place on the GenerationQ leadership programme with other participants in the same cohort, as well as across cohorts, with their coaches, in their action learning sets and with the wider faculty team. We would therefore like to thank and acknowledge every single leader who has taken part in GenerationQ for all they have done in their own work as a leader as well as all who have contributed to the stories told here.

Thirdly, we would like to thank the Health Foundation who commissioned, and have then funded, GenerationQ since 2009. It has given us as faculty a deeply satisfying source of work from which we ourselves have learned and gained enormously. It has also enabled us to get to know some truly fabulous, deeply committed people. Further thanks to Jennifer Dixon, Will Warburton and Frances Wiseman for their willingness to support our desire to disseminate some of the GenerationQ learnings more widely, by supporting the creation of this book and its companion volume, *Hope Behind the Headlines: Shifting culture in health and social care.* A particular thanks to Will for contributing to the thinking and writing of the opening chapters.

Project managing a group of senior leaders and authors with multiple commitments is not for the fainthearted, but Sue Jabbar has done a truly wonderful job, staying calm and being organised as versions of stories went to and fro. Our particular thanks to our faculty colleague, Pete Dudgeon, for helping to write some of the opening chapters and for supporting contributors in writing their own chapters. Likewise, Howard Atkins for supporting contributors who were often too busy to go it alone, and for offering kind words and help to us, the authors. Our thanks as well to Joy Furnival, a GenerationQ Fellow herself, for her support and the help she offered to the contributors.

Our thanks as well to our publishers, Libri, and to Paul Jervis for his confidence in what we had to offer and his patience as we worked out what the book was really about. James Baylay has added a wonderful visual element to the words which we believe really enhances the experience of reading the book.

Lastly our thanks to our families, friends and colleagues for putting up with the amount of time and energy it has taken to pull the book together, and for joining us in many conversations over the years. Our hope is that some of the inspiration and learning from this book will help our wonderful children see that they have choice as they enter the world of work and organisations. Each of them has been, and continues to be, our inspiration.

Contents

Preface

In my early days working in quality improvement, we often referred to the idea that 80 percent of quality problems are caused by the design of the system and 20 percent are attached to people issues. More recently I came across the following quote by Marjorie Godfrey from the Dartmouth Institute: "Improvement in healthcare is 20 percent technical and 80 percent human" (2012). For me it was a light bulb moment. Whilst the vast majority of the problems might be caused by system or process design issues, fixing those system or process issues requires the majority of the attention to be focused on the human aspects of change.

Recognising the systemic causes of quality problems prevents the inappropriate scapegoating of individuals, whilst ensuring the solutions focus on the issues that will make a difference. However, understanding that the majority of the challenges in addressing these systemic causes are attached, not to the technical application of quality improvement methods, but to the social aspects of change, is vital for ensuring effective implementation of those solutions. The real-life stories in this book illustrate how this dynamic plays out time and again in many different situations.

There is a saying that the effectiveness of a decision is equivalent to the quality of the decision multiplied by the commitment to implement it. This means that even the best solution in the world won't work if those tasked with implementing it don't believe in it. In this book you will consistently hear about the importance of taking the time to build the will for change in those who need to make the change.

Further, as long as a change will deliver an improvement, it is often better to go with a less than perfect solution that has the commitment of those implementing it, than an externally imposed ideal that has no local ownership. I was struck when I read through the stories how often those leading the work describe having to let go of their pre-formed ideas about what needs to happen, and instead move to a position of enabling others to come up with their own solutions. In doing so, these leaders are creating an environment where continuous improvement moves from a theoretical concept to a day-to-day reality.

However, that is not to say that the technical method doesn't matter. Deming, one of the gurus of quality improvement, reminds us that "hopes without a method to achieve them will remain mere hopes" (1982, p. 20). This book highlights the key quality improvement methods that are currently being used across health and social care services, and how they are being successfully applied to deliver significant improvements in care.

Core to all of the different methods is the concept of experimentation. Before I started on the GenerationQ programme, I tended to think of experimentation as something you applied to processes through, for example, the application of a plan, do, study, act (PDSA) cycle. However, GenerationQ taught me that experimenting with changes in how I approached and responded to social interactions can be equally important. And it is often the simplest of gestures that can make a difference: whether that be changing an initial response from a statement to an inquiring question; changing the layout of a room from chairs in a row to chairs in a circle; or simply taking the time to get to know something a bit more personal about the individuals we are working with day to day. The stories in this book all contain examples of small changes in gesture that had a far bigger impact than might be expected. They also highlight how much courage making those small changes can take.

As we celebrate 70 years of the NHS, and in Scotland, 50 years of the Social Work Scotland Act, we are facing some of the most significant financial and workforce challenges in our organisational histories. It is in this context that I recently came across the concept of the politician's fallacy: "We must do something (big). This is something (big). Therefore, we must do this".

I've added "big" onto this saying as, right now, the pressure on health and social care leaders to be seen to be making quick and large-scale change is enormous, even if that short-term action is going to make things worse in the longer term.

In reality, we do need some radical changes, but designing those from the centre is not the solution in a complex system where local contexts can derail even the best designed centralised initiative. Right now we need leaders with the courage to set a vision, and then enable those receiving and delivering services to work together with their wider communities to design and implement a new system of care that truly puts people at its centre. Whilst quality improvement methodologies alone won't deliver this, the stories in this book illustrate that, combined with authentic, reflective and politically astute leadership, they are an essential part of the solution.

However, the personal costs of leading improvement in this context are rarely shared, except in quiet moments amongst trusted colleagues and friends. For me, part of what makes this book and its companion, *Hope Behind the Headlines*, so important is that the authors have had the courage to tell the honest story of leading improvement, warts and all. It is hard work; more often than we like to admit it doesn't work, and sometimes it can be at considerable personal cost. Yet these improvement stories are some of the most inspirational I've ever read. In every one of them you read about individual leaders with a burning passion for making our health and care system better. And in their moments of success, you can't help but share a sense that the hard work was all worth it. If this is the future of leadership across health and social care in the UK, then I believe we are well placed to meet the challenges ahead.

Ruth Glassborow

Director of Improvement

Healthcare Improvement Scotland

Introduction

There can be few undertakings where high standards of quality are more important, to so many of us, than health and social care.

We all get ill at some point in our lives, or require support, and so do those around us. In the western world, we have come to expect that modern medicine can offer relief, and in some cases cure, for us, our families and friends when illness comes. Whilst most of us have experienced the skill, dedication and compassion of all those professionals involved in health and social care, so too, have some of us been on the receiving end of care which doesn't meet the highest standards, which involves delay or discomfort, where no one seems to be able to tell us what is going on, or where we feel alone and scared and nobody is there to reassure or just be with us.

The apparent answer to some of those shortcomings is to approach them with a view to changing them for the better, in other words to improve the quality of care. In this book we seek to understand the range of methods and approaches (the "toolkit") that already exists for quality improvement (QI), and to explore what it takes in practice to use these methods well, to bring about real and sustainable improvements in the quality of care.

Fundamentally we believe that good, sustainable and affordable improvement is possible, and is already happening in many places across the health and social care economy. Our optimism is not borne out of naïve beliefs or wishful thinking, but is the gift that we have been given by working with health care leaders over the years.

We, the authors, have many years of experience working in health and social care as organisation development practitioners and as leadership developers. The idea for writing this book emerged from our work as members of the faculty team in running and facilitating the Ashridge Masters in Leadership (Quality Improvement), funded by the Health Foundation and marketed as GenerationQ. The Q stands for Quality. Over the past eight years we have had the privilege and delight of working alongside one hundred and twenty-six ordinary, but at the same time remarkable, people. The participants, or Fellows as we call them, represent the full gamut of professions and skills needed to keep our health and care services running: nurses, allied health professionals, surgeons, clinicians, managers, paramedics, pharmacists, GPs, commissioners and policy makers. They all share a common purpose – to care well for patients and service users – as well as a desire to learn how to do it even better. It seemed a waste that only we were able to enjoy hearing what the GenerationQ Fellows were doing and learning as we read their assignments and Masters theses. Hence the idea of collecting and publishing some of their stories in this book.

In their stories, the Fellows share how they have each sought to improve the quality of care in their local environment. Each of them has chosen to put to the test one or more of the QI methods. They describe using these tools in earnest, often adapting them to meet the needs of their specific context. They also describe their own acts of leadership that go beyond the use of the tools, and share what they discover it takes to change things for the better in practice. The stories are of progress as well as some setbacks, of trying different approaches, of experimenting, of building organisational savviness, of getting to know themselves as leaders more deeply, of connecting with others, and being willing at times to be personally brave or vulnerable to improve things for the better.

The stories are written by the Fellows themselves, and they provide a rarely heard account of what it is like to lead in practice, "warts and all". Each story represents the perspective of one individual. They share their experiences of what actually happened when they were making moves to improve things for the better in their workplaces. The stories represent their truth, their learning, their inner dialogue about what they thought and felt, what they did and why. As we will all recognise, whenever any of us recount what happened at work, our accounts are always partial, as we choose what to share and what to leave out. The Fellows' stories are therefore not attempting to represent the truth, or provide a definitive answer, about "what actually happened" as an objective, scientific account.

Care has been taken to disguise the identity of the organisations and individuals within each story, to avoid any risk of unintentionally offending others. We trust that the stories evoke an empathetic and generous response in the reader, as they were written with the intention of being helpful to others who may be in similar situations. As the stories are written by the Fellows, expect the writing styles to be different and to reflect their individual voices.

The first three chapters set out some of the informing thinking and research about context, quality improvement methods and leadership to which Fellows are exposed on the GenerationQ programme. Each chapter also includes some short reflections and examples in the Fellows' own words, to illuminate how they applied these ideas and frameworks to their own experience as leaders. As you read the stories, you will see that many of the Fellows make reference to further theories or concepts that we have covered in the programme. We have included some of these in the appendices, to allow you, the reader, to dip into them as you wish. We hope that these ideas and frameworks are helpful for you, as well as giving you an insight into where the Fellows are coming from when you read their stories.

The book is organised in four sections:
- Section 1, *Framing*, comprises three chapters offering insight into what we mean by the toolkit and what is needed beyond it. You might choose to skip this section and turn straight to Section 2 where the stories begin, and perhaps then return to it later, if theory and research are not your main interest
- Section 2, *Experimenting,* comprises four story chapters each of which is a Fellow's story. The stories share a common theme of beginning the task of trying to improve quality, and choosing the time and the place where those experiments might be successful
- Section 3, *Engaging*, also comprises four story chapters. The theme here is that of recruiting others in the organisation to join the quality improvement endeavour.
- Section 4, *Committing*, comprises three story chapters which illustrate improving quality on a larger scale. In these stories three of our Fellows found fertile ground for their improvement efforts and had an impact which was organisation wide.

We end by offering our own closing reflections.

In addition, you may be interested in the companion volume, *Hope Behind the Headlines: Shifting culture in health and social care,* which also contains stories written by health and social care leaders.

Brian Marshall, Liz Wiggins, Janet Smallwood

February 2018

Framing

In this first section we offer three chapters that set out some of the informing thinking and research about context, quality improvement methods and leadership to which Fellows are exposed on the programme. The chapters also include some short reflections and illustrations in the Fellows' own words. Our intention in writing these chapters is to help you understand where the Fellows are coming from in their stories, and encourage your own reflection on what it means to lead quality improvement. It is also to set you up well for enjoying reading, and learning, from their stories.

In Chapter 1, *The Challenges of Leading Improvement,* we explore the context and complexity of the leadership task of improving quality in health and social care. We offer a way of thinking about the territory of actions and learning required of QI leaders, including those that go beyond the toolkit of QI approaches and methods to lead sustained improvement in the quality of care.

In Chapter 2, *The Toolkit,* we explore the contribution of the quality improvement (QI) methods and offer a "good enough" insight into the various theoretical approaches. Most of these approaches have been developed outside of health and social care, often in industry, with a view to reducing mistakes and thus improving quality at a reduced cost. Increasingly, however, these methods are being deployed extensively in health and social care, with somewhat mixed results. We get behind the individual theories to understand their underpinning thinking and assumptions, to use this to compare them, and to establish where they really differ and why.

In Chapter 3, *Beyond the Toolkit*, we begin to lay out why the toolkits examined in the previous chapter are useful but not sufficient. We examine how leading sustainable improvements in quality often requires leaders to pay attention to what we call four leadership domains. We explore what it means to be an effective relational leader, to be organisationally savvy, and to build effective relationships where leading QI is not a solo endeavour. We also examine how leaders need to understand themselves in more depth, to be aware of their own patterns of behaviour and what lies behind them. Many of the leadership moves or gestures that you will read about in the Fellows' stories – what they pay attention to and are aware of when working with the QI toolkits – arise from the approaches and insights shared in this chapter.

CHAPTER 1

The Challenges of Leading Improvement

A few words to start

Over the past eight years we have had the privilege and delight of working alongside one hundred and twenty-six ordinary, but at the same time remarkable, people. We, the authors, are lucky enough to be members of the faculty team running and facilitating the Ashridge Masters in Leadership (Quality Improvement), funded by the Health Foundation and marketed as GenerationQ. The Q stands for Quality. The participants, or Fellows as we call them, represent the full gamut of professions and skills needed to keep our health and care services running: nurses, allied health professionals, surgeons, physicians, managers, paramedics, pharmacists, GPs, commissioners and policy makers. They all share a common purpose – to care well for patients and service users – as well as a desire to learn how to do it even better.

We imagine that many of you reading this book will be leaders, or aspiring leaders, in either health or social care or the wider health economy. Our hope is that in reading these stories you will begin to recognise situations and to draw parallels with your own context, and that the stories will stimulate and encourage you to see new ideas and possibilities for your own role. We start from a position that the complexity and variety of patient care and patient need means that there is no silver bullet guaranteed to improve quality. We like the analogy that leading improvement is nearly as complicated an endeavour as raising a child (McCandless, 2008) – and we do not normally approach that challenge with a gap analysis or a Gantt chart! Instead we suggest leading quality improvement requires a similar attitude, engaging fully every day and being prepared to work with whatever arises. We believe that two key things can help you significantly:

1. Becoming familiar and comfortable with the tools which are available to help in improving quality (See Chapter 2, *The Toolkit*)
2. Knowing what else is needed and where else to place attention and effort in your role leading quality improvement (See Chapter 3, *Beyond the Toolkit*)

We hope that the Fellows' stories which then follow will give you ideas and insights into what can arise when leading improvement, and that reading about their choices will inspire and encourage you in your local context.

What do we mean by quality in health and social care?

Talk to any one of the Fellows and they all share the view that quality in health and social care can improve and, in some specific cases, needs to improve. This view is echoed by many observers and commentators. Don Berwick wrote;

> The most important single change in the NHS in response to this report [into Mid Staffs] would be for it to become, more than ever before, a system devoted to continual learning and improvement of patient care, top to bottom and end to end.

> (2013, p. 5)

Before considering what it takes to improve quality, it seems important to first examine what we mean by quality. Working with the Fellows and hearing their stories, it is apparent that quality means very different things to them and to different stakeholders. As one of the Fellows wrote in his application to join the programme:

> "Quality" is a ubiquitous word in the modern NHS. As part of my preparation for this piece, I asked every person I met over the course of a day – nurses, doctors, porters, and patients – what they understood by the word "quality". From a total of around forty people, I got almost as many different replies. An immediate challenge for anyone wanting to improve the quality of care we give in the NHS is ensuring everyone who is treated by and works in the NHS understands what is meant by this simple, short word.

In the first workshop of the programme, Fellows are invited to participate in a simple exercise which you might want to try for yourself with colleagues.

In small groups of three, they share stories of their own experience of either being a patient or being alongside a family member as a patient, describing the best aspects of the experience as well as the most troubling. Listening attentively, not just for the facts but for the emotions as well, they reflect together on what they have (re-)discovered is important to them. In effect, they are standing in the shoes of their own patients to (re-)see what quality means for them. The exercise is apparently simple and yet always profound. What surfaces is the importance of the effectiveness of medical care but this is just one factor amongst many. The value of being seen as a human being rather than a problem to be fixed is frequently mentioned, as is the importance of experiencing the human qualities of compassion, respect and empathy.

And of course, there are other stakeholders, in addition to patients, whose notions of quality need to be explored and taken into consideration when determining what needs to improve.

A widely used definition of quality comes from the Institute of Medicine (IOM) in the US, written by Don Berwick, who has also written about the need for culture change in the NHS. The IOM offer 6 *quality aims*, (Berwick 2002), stating that health care needs to be:

1. Safe
2. Effective
3. Patient-centred
4. Timely
5. Efficient
6. Equitable

One of the Fellows suggests that compassion merits addition as a seventh aim:

> *As part of my own work on this topic I reviewed the work of Don Berwick, in particular the Six Aims of Quality health care – safe, effective, efficient, timely, patient-centred and equitable. Whilst I am in no position to argue with these excellent aims I do wonder if we need to add a seventh – compassion. In my experience this can be the defining factor of what a patient perceives as "excellent care". Many complaints that I review show no deficit in the six aims outlined above but a staff member may have been unnecessarily rude or simply not cared enough and shown that in their behaviour. When we are at our most vulnerable it is these small acts of kindness, recognition of suffering – compassion – that can make all the difference. We work in a high pressure environment and it is understandable that tensions and stress can lead to a breakdown in compassion, indeed there is good evidence to support that compassion is the first thing to go in a stressful environment, but we must accept these "human factors" and learn from them and work on supporting our staff not to lose this vital quality as it is so important to delivering quality care.*

What seems important here is less the definitional accuracy of quality and more the recognition that there is a range of perspectives, and therefore there is a need to broker a good enough shared understanding when setting out to improve quality. As we consider further in Chapter 2, one of the challenges in using any QI method is that you can make no assumption that everyone shares the same understanding of quality, nor holds the same priorities about what needs to improve. This is undoubtedly because in health and social care, the context is complex and there are many stakeholders.

The challenges of leading quality improvement

The discussion above about what constitutes quality is, we believe, just one of the challenges facing a leader who is committed to improving quality in his or her context.

In examining challenges, we are mindful of twin risks: we do not want to naïvely ignore some of the challenges involved; neither do we want to amplify them so that it all feels too difficult. It therefore feels important to state up front that we believe that good, sustainable and affordable improvement *is* possible, and is already happening in many places across the health and social care economy. However, there are some unique circumstances in health and social care which ask a lot of leaders, and we have categorised these under six headings.

The six leadership challenges for quality improvement

When we designed the GenerationQ programme in 2010, we undertook extensive research, talking to leaders of quality improvement at different levels in a wide range of organisations. From this research, we identified six generic QI leadership challenges that are likely to be relevant to any leader of quality improvement, but will need to be uniquely understood and interpreted for each local context by each leader for themselves. These challenges are illuminated further in the stories later in the book.

1. Brokering sufficient multi-stakeholder participation and agreement

Most, if not all, efforts to improve quality involve multiple stakeholders, often with differing views on quality improvement priorities. Literally creating a map of the stakeholders can be a helpful initial step. They then need prioritising, as stakeholders will differ in terms of their power and influence. Some may represent different professional "tribes" such as nursing, medicine, surgery, or management. Others may represent different organisational entities, the latter increasingly the case when system-wide improvement is sought. The challenge for the QI leader is to broker sufficient agreement and buy-in between enough stakeholders so that initiatives are not derailed before they even begin.

One Fellow describes his challenge to broker agreement with the leader of a department:

> Tom was appointed just before me and was obviously keen to stamp his authority and show that he was capable of making change. My first dealings with him made me think that his approach to improving theatre utilisation was "like a bull in a china shop", and he always seemed to be "managing upwards". He wanted the changes that we were trying to make fully costed, and a business plan writing, which would take time I didn't have. Much later, when we'd abandoned the initiative, he told me he didn't feel I had recognised where he was coming from – "You never understood the pressure I was under as you weren't the one who had to go and explain this at Finance and Performance!"

We discuss in Chapter 3 some of the relational skills needed to meet these kind of challenges.

2. Leading others in complex change

There is increasing research evidence that a significant determinant of sustainable change is whether other people feel involved in, and part of, the change. However, a dominant style of leadership in health is that of "command and control", where change is imposed top down from on high, with the leader often feeling that they ought to sort things out, single-handedly.

Many of the leaders we work with talk of the burden of responsibility this brings, which can sometimes feel overwhelming. They talk of the pressures to "know," to behave as a heroic leader, feeling they should have an answer, even when there is no clear solution.

However, believing that as the leader you need to do it all yourself sets in motion a vicious cycle. The heroic model of leadership doesn't just set unreal expectations for the leader. It encourages followers to be passive onlookers, which can have a profound effect on culture and the sustainability of any quality improvement. This is expressed eloquently in *Living Leadership* (Binney et al 2012, p. 44), one of the books we ask the Fellows to read. The authors write:

> *The pressure of short term results, the sense of overload – too much to do and expectations that are confused or impossible to achieve … have led to two damaging and self-reinforcing patterns … The first is the leader staying distant from his people … the second is followers leaning back and refusing to take responsibility …Followers are let off the hook at the same time as leaders are impaled on it.*

For the rest of the organisation, the shadow side of seeing leadership as a heroic endeavour is that it encourages dependency, with little opportunity for staff to contribute, show initiative or to be engaged in improvement and change in any meaningful way.

A Fellow recounts his experience of not involving others in change:

> *When I was appointed to my consultant post, I joined what had been described by the Care Quality Commission (CQC) as a failing department. When I introduced myself to people, they would reply with phrases such as "Ah! You're here to sort us out!". I took on – and relished – the role of transformational, heroic leader, but this only led to the people I was working with passing more and more of the important decisions that needed to be made on to me. This then resulted in me seeing staff as being incapable of making decisions about not only the big crises, but increasingly menial matters.… As I took more and more control, this elicited a vicious circle where colleagues took less responsibility and placed more dependence on my decision-making. I decided what was best, made decisions, and then got frustrated when people didn't follow through. For example, when the CQC criticised the ward team hand-overs between shifts, I created an entirely new system to address their concerns. I did not liaise with the staff who would be using the system because I assumed they wanted me to fix it for them. I broke the connection between me and my team. Binney et al (2012, p. 37) say:*
>
> > *"If you treat others as the audience for your performance, then they will applaud from time to time – or throw rotten eggs – but they are unlikely to get up on stage and help you."*
>
> *My team threw rotten eggs at my ideas!*

This draws attention to the fact that *how* leaders approach the improvement effort, noticeably how they invite and encourage others to join them and to share responsibility, is vital.

3. Making informed choices about when and how to act

We encourage GenerationQ Fellows to be "choiceful". (We know the word doesn't exist, but we believe it should!) As a leader of QI, in your own context, there will be times for judging when to make a move and to be decisive and times when it is better to wait. This includes judging the appropriate scale and scope of any improvement intervention, as well as selecting an improvement method or approach, as will be explored in the next chapter.

For some QI leaders, particularly those without significant positional power, the way forward is often to start with small and discretely defined experiments that allow an opportunity for learning. These are often called Trojan Mice (Brown 1998) – experiments that are small, fast and operate below the radar. At the same time it is important to pay attention to the fact that making changes in one part of the system may well have unintended consequences in another part.

Sometimes interconnected steps in a process make it like squeezing a balloon – the part you are squeezing is thinner but everywhere else gets fatter to compensate. There are plenty of stories of this happening in practice. For example, if the focus of a hospital-based QI team is on quicker processing ("flow") of patients through hospital departments, patients could be put at risk of readmission unless there is also attention paid to what is needed to support their safety and recovery at home – which in turn may depend on the capacity of social care, community services and families to enable them to return to living independently.

As far as possible, quality improvement should be an improvement across the whole process not just in one part (Fillingham et al 2016). This is not to say that QI leaders need to work on the whole process at once, but rather that they need to be intelligent in understanding the links and the possible consequences of any changes made.

Working with the Fellows, we have also learned that a further trap is to believe there is a best or right improvement method to choose for each problem or endeavour. This can lead to procrastination, anxiety and the fear of getting it wrong. As you will read, most choices are made on a more pragmatic basis: What QI method and language is most widely shared in my context that I can build upon? What technical expertise already exists in the organisation for me to work with? What approach am I personally drawn to or have heard good stories about? What new method might have a chance of disrupting the dogma of "how things are" in my organisation?

4. Shifting the local culture to be more conducive to quality improvement

Shifting local cultures is the dedicated subject of the companion book to this, *Hope Behind the Headlines.* This challenge recognises that sometimes one of the first acts of leadership to encourage quality improvement is creating an environment where people feel able and willing to explore what is working well, what might be improved. Creativity and innovation are unlikely to emerge if there is fear, exhaustion and actual, or rumours of, bullying. As one of the story tellers says, "Shouting at a flower won't make it grow".

In some organisations, encouraging involvement from others, that is to say more bottom-up rather than top-down change, may itself be quite counter-cultural.

A Fellow reflects on his initial attempts to introduce Lean into an emergency department:

> *The success was never sustained and the good results we achieved felt as if they were entirely dependent on me having to work harder. Shifts when I was not there saw processes reverting back to how they used to be, and performance dropped again.*
>
> *In a senior ED team meeting preparing for a further attempt I was asked by my director to present what we had achieved and why I thought the idea had not gained any traction. I explained that if the idea was perceived as mine then it would be hard for anyone else to buy into the change. Whatever change we were going to make had to be owned by the staff. This prompted an awkward silence as this is so counter-cultural for our organisation which relies on top-down change. However, he acknowledged this was a novel strategy and one we should try. I breathed a sigh of relief.*

5. Sustaining self and others

As with raising a child, leading QI can bring moments of joy, fun and great personal satisfaction. It can also bring trials and tribulations: set-backs, conflict and sustained periods of living with uncertainty. Depending upon your own personal context and how much support you have, it can also be lonely. QI leaders therefore often face the challenge of developing their own personal resilience. This does not mean becoming tough or lacking in compassion. Rather, it involves getting to know yourself more, your "hooks and drivers", to understand what you personally need in order to be able to lead well over time. It requires learning to reflect and to develop a "third eye" to be able to notice what is going on for you and for others. This is explored further in Chapter 3.

Sustaining yourself may also involve building a local support network of a few people with whom you can reflect honestly about what is going on, and explore how you might be inadvertently contributing to some of the problems. It may involve working with a coach, being a member of an action learning set, or journalling. It may also be about remembering to pause and acknowledge progress alongside the difficulties, and to celebrate success. It may be ensuring that you and others have lives outside of work – time for family, taking exercise and so on.

6. Recognising and using the power of ambiguity and uncertainty

One of the ways that demands across the health and social care system manifest themselves in the local context can be in the pressure for quick fixes, for immediate solutions, with an impetus to close down disagreement and dissent or sweep it under the proverbial carpet. Yet one of the most powerful choices a leader of quality improvement can make is to recognise that there are different kinds of problems, and that some require living with and "holding" uncertainty. Let us look first at the different types of problems. We draw on the terminology of Rittel and Webber (1973) who refer to "tame" and "wicked" problems.

Tame problems

Tame problems are those which generally you or others have encountered before, and for which a solution or process is already in existence. The required action here is for leaders to identify the appropriate solution to the puzzle. However, it is important to recognise that tameness does not necessarily mean simplicity, or that a problem is easy to address – tame problems can be very complicated and thus the solution may also be very complicated. By-pass heart surgery, relocation, new product launch; these are all problems which have a solution and are therefore tame, even if that solution may be complicated and require skill to get right.

Wicked problems

Wicked problems do not have readily available solutions, either because they are novel, contextually and culturally specific or because they stubbornly resist any attempts at resolution. They tend not to have an end-point, and defining a condition where they are "solved" is normally not possible, or even desirable. Rather they tend to be characterised by better or worse developments. These kinds of problems are not often well suited to high planning, high control approaches. Instead the route forward is more exploratory, frequently using small experiments to try to see what works and what doesn't and to learn from them. This is the territory of many QI challenges, particularly when leading system-wide improvement or seeking to shift local cultures to be more conducive to improving quality of care.

To help think about the type of problems they are encountering, the GenerationQ Fellows have found what we call the Stacey Grid helpful (Stacey 1996). This grid represents the constant tension, which exists in all organisations or systems, between a desire for stability and the need for exploration and experimentation. In terms of change, relative stability would be characterised by a high level of agreement about what needs to happen, and a high degree of certainty in the environment. This is bottom left on the graph (Figure 1.1). This may be because the change or improvement in question is one that has been done before in a comparable context, hence the knowledge and confidence about what to do and how to do it. In the top right there is much more uncertainty in the environment and far less agreement about what to do or how to do it.

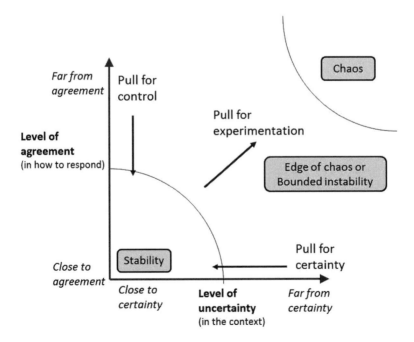

Figure 1.1: Zones of stability and instability. Adapted from the work of Stacey by Vanstone, Critchley and other Ashridge colleagues

The top right zone of this graph is seen as chaotic. In this way of looking at organisations, messiness and uncertainty are acknowledged and even perceived as creative spaces with multiple possibilities for the new to emerge. An executive director at Marks and Spencer was overheard saying in a senior strategy meeting, "It's really good we're confused about this. If we thought we knew what we were doing here we'd cock it up. We need some uncertainty to give us room to think". Similarly the CEO of Shell USA told his leaders at their conference "The world is a messy place. If we want to stay on top of the corporate ladder, we must plunge into the mess. We must learn to work with the mess" (Wiggins and Hunter 2016, p. 19).

The Fellows use the grid as a prompt to reflect upon the nature of the QI challenge they face: Is there a ready answer? Should they know the way forward or is more exploratory work needed? Often, thinking about QI in this way helps them push back against expectations of heroic leadership. Equally, improvement requires people to think and act differently, and whether or not people are willing to do so is also neither predictable nor certain. The challenge for the QI leader is to not close down the uncertainty too soon, not to rush for answers or tell people what to do, even as anxiety increases. Rather, it is to stay with the uncertainty as new and creative possibilities for action begin to emerge.

These six generic challenges are designed as a guide; each will need to be interpreted and made real and personal for each leader. However, we trust that they map out some of the territory that perhaps you have already experienced. We hope that you feel similar to one of the Fellows who said:

> *The GenerationQ leadership challenges were central to me deciding to apply for GenQ. My immediate reaction was "at last someone understands". They felt very reassuring.*

The macro context – additional challenges

Talk to almost anyone working in health and social care, and people describe the current macro context as particularly tough. Leadership experts also suggest that leading the improvement of quality in the context of health care is arguably one of the most challenging areas of modern leadership (Gregory et al 2012). Resource constraints, technological advances, increasing patient demands and the pervasive impact of party politics, election cycles and policy changes all contribute to the health care context being frequently described as **V**olatile, **U**ncertain, **C**omplex and **A**mbiguous (VUCA), using Stiehm and Townsend's (2002) ugly but succinct acronym.

It therefore feels important to acknowledge some of the factors we hear as contributing to this challenging macro context, much of which will undoubtedly be familiar to you. We mention these because it is important not to deny current reality when leading improvement, and because the Fellows' stories are, we hope, evidence that improvement can be achieved despite this.

The widening gap between demand for care and available funding

A common theme we hear from health leaders in the programme, as well as in the mainstream and medical press, is the constant pressure for further efficiency savings *at the same time* as increasing demand for services. The NHS in England, for example, has responded to the pressures by aiming to make £22 billion of efficiency savings by 2020 (Lafond et al 2016), whilst the reality is that by the end of 2016, 57 percent of Trusts were in deficit (Charlesworth et al 2017). In the 2015 Comprehensive Spending Review, the government committed additional funding for health in England of £4.5 billion by 2020/21, but this equates to an increase in NHS funding of just 0.7 percent per year in real terms. This is the lowest increase since the creation of the NHS in 1948 and comes at a time when demand for health care services is estimated to be increasing at around four percent a year, and public funding for adult social care has fallen in real terms. This creates an inevitably challenging climate in which to work, with constant uncertainty and anxiety about funding levels and availability of resources to deliver existing services, let alone improve them. It also means that all too often quality improvement is the espoused agenda, but what is experienced "on the ground" is the singular pressure to cut costs, at all costs.

The demand for quick fixes

It would be all too easy to lay the blame for short-termism at the feet of politicians who need to be re-elected, or senior executives who want to keep their jobs. Yet it is of course more complicated than that, and at least in part a consequence of the significant gap between resources and demand. All of us, as a society, are perhaps also colluding in avoiding the difficult choices about what we are collectively prepared to pay for and how. Leaders in health and social care are increasingly telling us about the impact and perils of short-term thinking. One leader who tells the story of doing fabulous work in improving the quality of the patient experience doubts that she would now be given the time and space to achieve what she has in recent years. Another says,

In my view, we don't appoint poor leadership teams, it's just that we don't let them do the job they need to do in the way they need to do it. We are obsessed with turnaround and quick fixes and when the fix doesn't happen fast enough we change the leadership team. To me, it's a form of madness.

The challenge of finding and keeping good people

The likelihood is that, wherever you work, there are vacancies that you are having trouble filling. The causes and indeed the solutions are complex. The impact on those trying to lead in health and social care to maintain service levels, let alone improve and innovate, is significant. One leader described the impact in his context:

There is a steady stream of junior doctors leaving the country to practise elsewhere or leaving medicine altogether. 51% of Scottish foundation doctors left medicine after their second postgraduate year in 2016. This, along with other factors, has led to a significant shortage of consultants and GPs. These shortages are felt everywhere but in small district general hospitals like ours it is felt even more. We are currently sitting with 30 percent consultant vacancies and nearly 40 percent of GP positions unfilled. This has led to an unprecedented reliance upon locum doctors who, recognising an opportunity, have slowly increased their rates. We have some locum doctors earning a fortune each a week. They work hard and yet this is hard to stomach when the constant refrain from senior management is that there "is no money" and that we all need to "tighten our belts" and change how we work to save money. We have a £20 million CRES (cash releasing efficiency scheme) target but an £11 million locum spend. It is understandable that our permanent staff get frustrated and wish to know that we are doing everything that we can to recruit more permanent staff.

The expectation placed upon leaders

Leaders sometimes talk about the combination of the first three factors – not enough money, not enough time and not enough people – as a perfect storm, leading to overstretch, stress and workplace-related illness. In addition to this, the expectations placed upon them about how to lead and how much power and authority they have can feel at odds with what is needed to lead improvement. The norm in the health service continues to emphasise heroic leadership styles, with calls to leaders from those in authority to be in control and to have the answers; for "grip", "pace" and "strong leadership" over the more inclusive, relational style that complex improvement problems call for.

The nature of power and authority held by leaders is also often far from clear and needs to be negotiated, particularly when leadership requires collaboration across professional "tribes", such as between clinicians and managers, and, at a system level, between multiple regulators, commissioners, providers and policymakers.

The art of responding well to this complexity and apparent lack of clarity can be compromised by leaders' lack of development. Clinicians, for example, are highly trained individuals, but many have received little or no management or leadership development. Often, they pursue their management objectives through intuition or a style developed from observing others. Sometimes this can be effective, but can also lead to leadership with little awareness about impact upon others, or indeed self. You might well be choosing to read this book because you have recognised this for yourself.

Summary

In this chapter we have explored what is meant by quality and recognise that, while there is agreement that improvement in quality is needed in health and social care, it is a complex and challenging landscape in which to lead. In this context, knowledge of the QI methods and approaches – the toolkit – is necessary and yet not sufficient.

In the next chapter we examine some of this leadership territory in more depth, beginning with the toolkit of available QI methods and approaches.

CHAPTER 2

The Toolkit

Introduction

In this chapter, we consider the broad principles and approaches of five methods used to improve health and social care. Our intent here is to provide a high-level tour of quality improvement approaches that are commonly used, to bring them to life. It is not to offer an in-depth guide to each and every improvement approach. Our assumption is that, like the Fellows who apply to the GenerationQ programme, you want to lead improvement and choose thoughtfully between methods, without being totally immersed in the detail. We therefore look at the underlying philosophy and ideas that underpin each approach; we illustrate the similarities and differences between the methods, and aim to give you sufficient reference points and orientation so you can enjoy the contributors' stories if the technical domain is relatively unfamiliar territory for you.

There are three other observations we wish to make here.

Firstly, the title of this book, *Beyond the Toolkit*, already declares our hand, but let us be explicit. In our experience, working with senior health and social care leaders on the GenerationQ programme, we know that a good set of quality improvement methods and tools is absolutely necessary in making improvements, but on their own, we believe they are not sufficient. The additional leadership skills required are contextual, relational and personal leadership. The importance of context was introduced in Chapter 1. Relational and personal leadership are explored in more depth in Chapter 3.

Secondly, quality improvement approaches are often referred to by the collective noun of the "improvement sciences". The term "scientific" may convey a certain credibility and status; data is often collected and evidence used to guide improvement efforts and monitor progress. However, in our experience, labelling these approaches scientific can be misleading. It can suggest that the methods can be applied objectively (at least among those who have a positivist scientific view of the world), minimising the vital requirement to notice and adapt to the local context. It can ignore the messiness of organisational life, and the likely emergence of power, politics, ego and resistance that accompany any changes, whether or not they are described as improvement. The term scientific also suggests the possibility of right and wrong answers; that there can be guarantees; that all that is required is to learn a method well and then apply it rigorously. The shadow side of calling improvement approaches scientific is that it may therefore unwittingly set them up as panaceas, idealising their potential to solve organisational issues and thus creating unrealistic expectations. When things then don't go quite to plan, as inevitably they don't, individuals may blame the method, or berate themselves or others for "not doing it correctly". This is why we delight in the notion of *good* practice as a source of learning and ideas but avoid the concept of best practice which suggests that there is a silver bullet – that all that is needed is to "plug and play" and all will be sorted. Rather than using the term improvement science, we thus prefer the phrase improvement methods or approaches.

Thirdly, listening to the experiences of the health and social care leaders with whom we work, we notice that sometimes people have had a negative experience with a particular method. It is then easy to dismiss or undervalue this approach. At the other end of the spectrum, there are those who have become so enthusiastic and deeply wedded to a particular method that their almost messianic zeal can leave others feeling alienated and disengaged. Our encouragement is to keep an open mind as you discover the thinking and principles that underpin different methods. In writing this chapter, we are not attempting to advocate one method over another, but to provide a tour of the territory. We recognise that labelling approaches – whilst necessary – may help to breed competition between the advocates of different schools of thought, but we are struck more by the shared historical origins, commonalities and synergies between methods than by divergence.

In our exploratory tour of the terrain, which we refer to as the technical leadership domain, we consider the following methods:

1. Lean
2. Theory of Constraints (TOC)
3. Institute for Healthcare Improvement (IHI) Model for Improvement
4. Experienced Based Co-Design (EBCD)
5. Appreciative Inquiry (AI)

1. Lean

Lean has provoked considerable interest in health care in the UK for more than a decade. It is an approach that originated in Japan, developing out of the Toyota Production System, and is now generally known simply as Lean. Toyota were seeking ways of improving how they built cars efficiently and in a way which enabled them to respond to changing customer demands. They studied mass production in Ford, and concluded that they need to shift the focus of the manufacturing engineer from individual machines and their utilisation to the flow of the product through the total process. Lean is often summarised as consisting of the following five principles:

 i. See what we do at work as a set of processes, all with the aim of adding value to the end user, be that a customer, service user or patient

 ii. Investigate and map out those processes. Distinguish between steps in those processes which add value, and those which don't

 iii. Seek to make each process flow without interruption in the best way possible. Avoid unnecessary steps, delays or waiting

 iv. Let the end user pull the process when they need it ("just in time"). Don't do things before they are needed, or in large batches

 v. Never stop trying to improve every process. Improvement should be forever

Sitting underneath these principles are two key aspects of Lean: standardisation and the elimination of waste. Standardisation means establishing a single way for everyone to undertake a process and forms the solid basis from which improvements are then made. Without an agreed standard, there is a danger that people may not be making improvements from the same starting point. I may improve my process, but if you already do it a different way, my improvement may not apply or may have a different effect. The elimination of waste involves critically examining processes in order to take out anything which does not add value (see Principle ii above). Let us look at these two aspects in more detail, as we find that they give Fellows on the programme a deeper understanding of the philosophy which sits behind the Lean methodology.

a) Standardisation

Taiichi Ohno, one of the creators of the Toyota Production System and thus one of the originators of Lean, declared that standardisation is the foundation of the Toyota Production System. Yet there are some common misconceptions about standardisation and how it is best applied within a health and social care setting. For instance, when we talk to Fellows about standardisation, some look concerned, and tell us that clinicians in their context are very resistant to any notions of moving away from individualised patient care. However, as Don Berwick, a leading authority on health care quality and improvement in both the US and the UK said,

> Standardisation and individualisation of care are not a contradiction. We make absolutely reliable what we need to make reliable. Avoid variation that does not add value to the individual. We are talking about mass customisation, as Taiichi Ohno said: When waste is at a minimum, the needs of the individual can be seen more clearly.
> (Don Berwick, 22 April 2010)

So, in talking about standardisation, we are not talking about being unresponsive to the needs of the individual. Rather, the argument is that by making an approach reliable, it is then possible to see individual needs more clearly.

It is significant that in Toyota, standards have traditionally been written in pencil. "So what?" you might be saying. "Who cares if standards are written in pencil, pen, or invisible ink?" However, it does matter for the simple reason that *everyone* knows how to use a pencil. There is no need to be computer literate, so anyone can write standard operating procedures, documenting "the best that you know today, but which is to be improved tomorrow ...", as Henry Ford said. In addition, the beauty of using a pencil is that it can easily be erased and a new, better way described.

This contrasts strongly with the way standards operate within the Health Service. There are many types: nationally agreed checklists, clinical best practices, local policies and so on. Some of these (in particular checklists) have proved their worth in helping to ensure there is a common approach to many different procedures and practices. However, none of these really capture the nature of what Ohno meant because he believed standards should be locally owned, even where informed by national or international good practice. The leaders on GenerationQ, often remark upon the marked absence of local ownership – for example the laminated list describing who can do which procedure, to assist those booking patients onto an array of procedures, is probably not owned by the department using them, but by those in greater authority. Because work content and personnel change so quickly, the moment these documents are printed and laminated they can become nothing more than glossy clutter, only briefly achieving their intended purpose. As these laminated standards rarely reflect operational reality, the outcome is often the opposite of that intended: overworked managers frequently interrupted with questions such as: "Whose list should I book this patient onto?" – a question which undermines the confidence of the person having to ask and drains the time of the expert.

So a pencil is just a metaphor: one which represents local ownership of a process which is always up to date and always the best method. (This is very different from the idea of best practice, where something that has worked in another context is transplanted everywhere. Here best method is developed and owned locally.) This brings us to the next natural step: now that the best method for the current context has been captured, what happens when an improvement is discovered?

Quality, safety and speed may all be features of what is described as the best method to date. We all know people who have a knack for developing effective shortcuts, often finding quicker and more effective ways of doing something, compared with their colleagues. Standardisation should promote the sharing of these methods: this is the standardisation intended by Taiichi Ohno. Standard work and standardisation, as understood in this way, ensure consistent high-quality patient care. It is not a policy document written once and only updated when inspectors are coming.

A host of other useful ideas follow from this basic concept of standardisation. If a standard process for patient care can be written (in pencil!), local ownership is possible. There is a basis for reliability because a group of people have recorded the best way they collectively know how to do this process. They also know how many people it takes and for how long to do this process, not as a route to staff cuts, but as a way of ensuring the process is done reliably. There is consistency in patient care.

Just as importantly, standardisation provides a platform or launch point for further improvement. There may be a communications area or a daily huddle. The latter is a short meeting, with people standing up to encourage succinctness, where there are conversations to review how things are working and what improvements could be made. There may be a desire to spend time studying the current processes to improve them, so there is an opportunity to use a tool called Value Stream Mapping. To ensure the process is the best it can be, any wasteful steps will need to be removed. To identify and eliminate different types of waste (referred to as Muda in the Toyota Production System), there may be a Plan, Do, Check, Act cycle of experimentation. Or we may choose to focus on an issue through the use of an A3 sheet, which seeks to scope, diagnose and suggest countermeasures all on one sheet of paper. These tools all sit under the umbrella of Lean.

b) Eliminating waste and continuous flow

The authors of a recent report focus on the need and opportunity throughout the OECD, including the UK, to reduce waste and thereby improve effectiveness and value for money, without detriment to other quality criteria:

> *Across OECD countries, a significant share of health care system spending, and activities are wasteful at best, and harm our health at worst. One in ten patients in OECD countries is unnecessarily harmed at the point of care. More than 10 percent of hospital expenditure is spent on correcting preventable medical mistakes or infections that people catch in hospitals... Meanwhile the market penetration of generic pharmaceuticals – drugs with effects equivalent to those of branded products but typically sold at lower prices – ranges between 10-80% across OECD countries...Strategies to reduce waste can be summed up as i) stop doing things that do not add value; and ii) swap when equivalent but less pricey alternatives of equal value exist. (2017)**

Waste also matters to patients, especially the waste that comes with waiting.

> *Every day is a really long day when you're either waiting to see the consultant, waiting for the results, waiting for a scan. It's another sleepless night, another day of worry. It's that uncertainty. It's the not knowing that's really hard to deal with. (Extract from a BBC interview with Nikki, an oesophageal cancer sufferer, Oct 2017)*

One of the most difficult experiences of people using health and care services is waiting. Waiting targets were introduced within the NHS in the 1990s and have had some positive impacts as well as unintended consequences in terms of behaviour. There are cases of people being employed to check breach lists (the clock should have stopped for that patient!), opening observation wards to "admit" people therefore stopping the clock on the four-hour A&E wait, and, dare we say, "gaming" where the computer system used for reporting doesn't match reality, in an effort to hit targets. All of this is understandable – "Every system is perfectly designed to get the results it gets" is a commonly heard QI phrase[†] – yet these actions detract from the target's intention: to encourage the reduction in waiting times.

Viewing this through a Toyota lens, reducing waiting times comes down to two fundamental concepts:
  i) Removing the delays that are designed in, which often requires reducing batch sizes
  ii) Achieving sufficient capacity to deal with demands

Both these ideas are encapsulated within the concept of "Just in Time". This

---

*   The UK is at the top of the OECD league table in 2015 for the market penetration of lower cost and effective generic drugs (OECD, 2017)

†   Source disputed; may have been Edwards Deming, Don Berwick or Paul Batalden

suggests just enough product at just the right moment in time to satisfy customer demands. It also, less explicitly, includes a concept that has significant implications for tackling the delays experienced in health care: that of continuous flow.

The principle of continuous flow essentially means that all value-added actions should happen, without delay in any product or service delivery. Now, for some medical conditions, at certain stages, time without action is exactly what *is* needed. However, in the vast majority of instances, as described by the patient above, waiting is the enemy of good-quality health care: condition deterioration, increased likelihood of infections, impacts on mental health and emotional wellbeing because of worry and not knowing. In many instances, applying the principle of continuous flow could provide part of the solution.

To see the benefits of continuous flow it is helpful to consider the opposite: batch thinking. If your GP waits until the end of the day to send on your referral, batching it with her other referrals, you have waited up to a day. If consultants triage new referrals on a weekly basis, you have typically waited half a week. If a ward round is conducted once a day, there will be patients ready for discharge who have not been seen yet, many of whom have been waiting, ready for discharge, for up to half a day.

When you start to see batching, you see it everywhere. Batching is so ingrained in our nature, tackling it requires what Womack and Jones refer to as, "rearranging our mental furniture" (2003).

And even if the negative impact of batching is recognised, lurking in the back of many people's minds there is likely to be a running script that goes something along the lines of "they haven't got capacity do deal with it now, so however much I rush it to them ('them' being the next person/service in the chain) they won't deal with it anyway, because they have a backlog". That self-talk is probably correct. Reducing waiting to increase waiting elsewhere is often futile. This is where the second concept comes in: achieving sufficient capacity. This is often seen as the Holy Grail of health care provision, and there are further two simple concepts underpinning it: demand and capacity.

Let's take demand. It is widely reported that demands on the health and social care system are at an all-time high due to a growing, ageing population. Moreover, the needs of individuals are becoming more complex, more frequently requiring multidisciplinary input. Greater capacity is required to deal with this. This leaves us with two fundamental choices: increase resources, or improve productivity (perhaps both).

GenerationQ Fellows have commonly found that in the NHS organisations where they work, demands are not generally understood well enough to make effective decisions over capacity. At an overall level demands may be known: how many attendances at A&E, how many referrals for different specialties. However, this does not provide the granularity required to design and plan services. More detail is required.

Take Endoscopy. It is not sufficient to know how many colonoscopy referrals are received. Clinicians also need to know how many require polyp removal. Why is this important? Because demand information needs to be at the same level of detail as that used to design services. For instance, the question "How many clinicians do we need skilled enough to perform Polyp removal?" can only be answered by knowing the number of these cases seen. Becoming better at understanding the nature of demands is the first step towards solving some of these capacity issues.

Let's hear from one GenerationQ Fellow who applied Lean thinking to understand demand and capacity:

> I had never looked at how many patients attended each hour of the day or how that varied throughout the week. Neither had I looked at when our surges in activity occurred or whether our staffing was adequate to meet variations in demand. [As it transpired] our busiest time of day was consistently between 11:00 to 18:00hrs. I decided to look at our hourly capacity to assess patients for each hour. This demonstrated how long the queue was going to be each hour.
>
> It was apparent that in terms of queue size our busiest time of day was indeed the evening, but this appeared to be due to our inability to conquer the surge in demand that occurred mid-morning and we struggled to regain control until demand naturally dropped at midnight. Not only had I come up with a reason for why we struggled every day, but I also had data that I could use to explain to others why the system needed to change. I felt a combination of emotions: pride in what I had achieved, but also slight embarrassment that I (or my colleagues) had never thought of doing this before.

Matching capacity to demand is crucial and fundamental to the application of Lean thinking.

Capacity is based upon two elements: how much resource you have and what tasks those resources (human and otherwise) are undertaking. Ohno described tasks as containing both value-added activities and wastes. If you are a consultant, how much of your day is spent waiting for patients to be ready? If you are a mental health professional, how much of your day is spent typing notes? In short, how can we identify wastes which can be addressed, in an effort to improve productivity? Ohno defined seven wastes, which were activities that consumed resource but added no value. But

Ohno's wastes were based on production. What are the wastes you see in health care? Inappropriate referrals? DNAs? Another Fellow wrote:

> Having both the process map and the demand map allowed us to analyse our processes. It was clear that not all our steps added value. For example, triage is a step which essentially has been created to risk-stratify the demand. Although analgesia may be provided where necessary, patients are ultimately told how long they have to wait depending on how ill they are. This results in relatively well patients waiting the longest time to see the clinician. So, the "worried well" frequently have to wait several hours for a two-minute consultation. This results in poor patient satisfaction and leads to overcrowding.

A characteristic of a Lean organisation is often described as being a place where the overwhelming majority of staff arrive at work each morning excited by the possibility of removing/reducing more waste from their day to day work. Another Fellow introduced Lean into his ED department and talked to nurses about their experiences:

> "I love it," said Zoe. "I can see the patients getting the right care and I am proud knowing I have done a good job."

> Hannah said "Being able to take pride in your work is something new for me. I have worked in this ED for five years, and this is the first time I look forward to coming to work and feel that I have done a good job."

> "It's still hard work," added Zoe. "When you've been in ED you know about it, but somehow it feels more organised which makes it less stressful."

2. Theory of constraints in health and social care

"Where on earth do we start with our improvements?" was an insightful question asked by Eli Goldratt, the thinker associated with Theory of Constraints. His observation was that in organisations there was often a deep sense of being overwhelmed when trying to design and manage processes. He argued that often there is neither the time nor the resources available to attempt this. We also believe very few isolated improvements have a positive impact on the system performance overall, given that there is always one part of the system, the most constrained part, that dictates the success of the system. In his book, *The Goal: A process of ongoing improvement* (2004), he therefore advocates working on the biggest system constraint first, through the following process:

    i.   Identify the system's constraint

ii. Decide how to exploit the system's constraint (make sure it keeps running)

iii. Subordinate everything else to the above decision (don't get distracted by other priorities)

iv. Elevate the constraint (increase its capacity)

v. If, in the previous step, a constraint has been broken, go back to the first step

So how are constraints identified? In classic Theory of Constraints application, it is about knowing which part of the system has the greatest negative mismatch between its capacity and the demands placed upon it. This might suggest that again there is a need to know the demands and capacity of each part of the system. That is certainly one way, but Goldratt, and later Alex Knight in his book, *Pride and Joy* (2014), argue that the largest queue is often just before the system's constraint, so this can be a strong indicator of where the constraint is. It is just like on a motorway where a big queue is a sure sign of an accident or roadworks up ahead.

One of our Fellows (a surgeon) explains his analysis of his context and his identification of "the constraint":

> *It was my assumption that, because it seems that the biggest queue in the patient pathway is before the operation, once it has been checked that the patient is fit for surgery, then the actual process of putting the patient through their operation in theatre must be the constraint. Therefore exploiting the constraint ... should allow greater flow through the pathway, and so reduce waiting times for patients.*

However, sometimes the constraint requires further investigation. To take an example, a recent report by NHS Improvement highlighted a huge amount of lost operating theatre time, the equivalent of 280,000 additional non-emergency operations. They stressed the effect this wasted capacity has on waiting times. The level of late starts and early finishes was defended by surgeons, who argued that it's often futile to get an extra patient into theatre because of the bed-stock situation. The argument went that a lack of social care beds was blocking patient hospital beds and therefore, even if theatre performance could be increased, those patients would have nowhere to go. So, to the surgeons, the constraint wasn't theatre, it was further downstream and therefore improvements to theatre utilisation would be largely futile.

A number of Trusts have adopted a process for regularly collecting data to indicate which resource, or lack of resource, is causing the greatest delays to the greatest number of patients. Informed by this, improvement efforts are then prioritised.

On the programme we introduce the Theory of Constraints to leaders by playing the Dice Game. Fellows have then used it with staff, as described in Chapter 7. The Dice Game consists of passing a number of counters, representing patients, from one participant to another, simulating the flow of patients through a system. The game shows very quickly and graphically what happens in a system, and how far apart the theoretical capacity and reality often are. In essence the process only ever flows as fast as its slowest step, no matter how hard everyone else tries to work.

3. The Model for Improvement and the Institute for Healthcare Improvement (IHI)'s approach

With Lean and Theory of Constraints, discussion is around improving flow, reducing waiting times, reducing waste and improving quality. Neither has the adoption and spread of *clinical* best practice at its core. Given that a fundamental purpose of any health care system is to be clinically effective, this opens up an incredibly important further area for exploration. A common assumption of both of Lean and the Theory of Constraints approaches in health care is that, predominantly, the "product", that is to say clinical practice, is designed to meet the needs of the patient or service user; the task therefore is to deliver this in the most efficient and effective way. The Institute for Healthcare Improvement, often referred to as IHI, have developed an approach to test changes to clinical (and non-clinical) practice and to spread those changes, their Model for Improvement (originally developed by Associates in Process Improvement*). The basis for their model originates with Walter Shewhart, an American physicist, engineer and statistician, sometimes known as the father of statistical quality control. He developed a way of using experimentation to move towards a solution and created the Plan-Do-Study (originally Check) -Act cycle. Also used in Lean, the PDSA cycle encourages us to try out changes and carefully observe the impact, before incorporating learning into the next cycle.

In taking Shewhart's Plan-Do-Study-Act cycle and incorporating three initial questions (Figure 2.1), the IHI has popularised a method which has gained such traction in UK health care that it is often seen as synonymous with Quality Improvement (QI). Indeed, many Trusts have the Model for Improvement at the core of their QI strategy. Its power is in its simplicity, with many clinical and non-clinical staff using it as a helpful framework for improvement.

---

*   For more information about Associates in Process Improvement visit http://www. apieweb.org

Model for Improvement

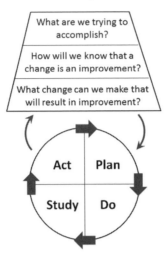

Figure 2.1. Source: Langley et al, The Improvement Guide (2009)

The model gives health care staff a way of testing a change on a small scale, so that a workable improvement can be arrived at before rolling out on a larger scale.

The first question – "What are we trying to accomplish?" – encourages staff to be clear about the aim of the cycle and to challenge the project if it is too vague or overly large and ambitious.

The second question – "How will we know if the change is an improvement?" – invites staff to think, before they begin, about how they will measure the results of their cycle, and implicitly to identify what success will look like.

The third question – "What changes can we make that will result in improvement?" – seeks to shape the overall change concept which is to be tested. These initial three questions quickly scope the project and begin the process of thinking about the change that could be used.

The Plan-Do-Study-Act cycle consists of setting up the test (plan), running the test (do), reflecting on and observing what happens (study), and finally noting what you would do differently next time (act).

In addition, driver diagrams (Figure 2.2) are frequently employed to establish target areas for improvement. Driver diagrams seek to understand what might be contributing to the problem that needs to be solved, and thus to generate ideas for change which will address some of the underlying causes ("drivers"). By breaking the overall problem down in this way, it enables even complex issues to be addressed through a combination of a number of small tests of change.

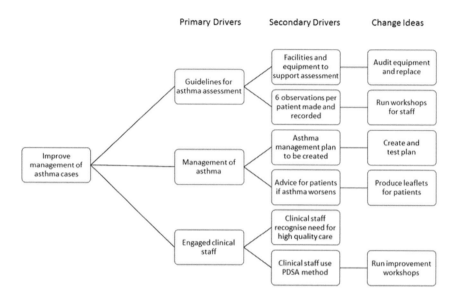

Figure 2.2. Fictional example of the use of Driver Diagrams

Here's a GenerationQ Fellow in a mental health organisation talking about his experience with the IHI model for improvement:

> Working with one inpatient ward team, we arranged to meet and begin to develop our driver diagram, or our theory of what makes violence more likely to happen. This was a great way to engage a team with the issue and hear what they thought were the main contributing factors within their environment. While the main aim – reducing violence – was relatively straightforward to define and describe, the primary drivers were less so and required a good deal of thought and engagement with those who work in the clinical area. We had expected a decrease of perhaps 20-25 percent in violence but instead, over six months we saw this decrease by an astonishing 90 percent.

Joseph Juran, Walter Shewhart and Edwards Deming are often cited as originating some of the methods and thinking in use in QI today (in Lean as well as the IHI). The IHI have explored ways of incorporating more of Juran's trilogy: Quality Improvement, Quality Control and Quality Planning (Scoville et al 2016). This is an interesting development, given that both

Toyota and the IHI are heavily influenced by the thinking of Juran, Deming and Shewhart. This is an example of some of the boundaries between Lean and IHI approaches becoming less distinct, perhaps helpfully so, as will be discussed later.

4. Experienced Based Co-Design (EBCD)

Most who work in health care, whatever their role, consider themselves to be patient-focused and wanting to help people. Patients or service users are, after all, the reason health care organisations exist. And yet the Fellows describe how they sometimes feel as though the health and social care systems conspire against staying focused on those very people who should benefit from them.

Putting user experience at the heart of design has been prevalent in the service industry for decades, and was adapted for use in a health care context by Bate and Robert (2006). Some Trusts have decided to have an entire team dedicated to facilitating improvement through engaging staff and patients in equal measure. The first steps involve gathering experiences from patients and staff through in-depth interviewing, observations and group discussions, in order to identify key "touch points". These are moments which were emotionally significant, and evoked either positive or negative feelings. A short, edited film is created from the patient interviews. The notion of patient stories as data is thus central to EBCD. The film is shown to staff and patients, conveying in an impactful way how patients experience the service. Staff and patients are then brought together to explore the findings and to work in small groups to identify and implement activities that will improve the service or the care pathway.

Areas for improvement are then jointly developed and monitored for four to six months. The emphasis here is on joint working – co-creating and designing the experience that is best for the patient.

With other approaches, whether or not staff and/or patients are involved is more heavily dependent on the personal preferences, as well as relational skills, of those leading the improvement. There is certainly growing evidence of EBCD being deployed in a range of settings from emergency departments, radiography, and mental health, to the design of care in wards for the frail and elderly, motivating staff and engaging patients in creating tangible and sustained improvements (see for example Springham and Robert 2015).

5. Appreciative Inquiry (AI)

The improvement methods described so far tend to start by looking at what went wrong, identifying problems and critical incidents. The last method we explore here, and on GenerationQ, offers an alternative to this deficit-based view and is underpinned by the principle that "...to discover and theorise about the life-giving properties of organisations – what is happening when they are operating at their best – is more likely than problem solving to lead to innovation". The key idea is that the more we focus on what went wrong, the more that problems and difficulties become all we see. They become our reality.

Appreciative Inquiry was developed in the 1980s by David Cooperrider and colleagues at Case Western Reserve University. They were working on a consulting project for the patient hotel at the Cleveland Clinic. Cooperrider and his team noticed how stuck in despair staff were when talking about the problems, so took them to visit a high-quality, high-performing hotel nearby, but with the instruction that employees could ONLY ask about what led to the hotel's success and explore what enabled them to keep performing well. Once the employees had become trained and practised in asking positive, rigorous inquiry questions, they were invited to turn their attention to their own hotel but again, to only identify what was working well, looking for sources of strength and success. Attempting to solve problems was not allowed.

Two features to draw attention to with this method:
   i.   The focus is on asking questions rather than stating positions and opinions
  ii.   There is a shift from problem solving and deficit talk to an appreciative stance

Deficit-based statements would be "I think the problem with this is…", "We should have done it differently", "This won't work because…." or "We've tried that before". Deficit-based questioning would be "What is the main problem?" "Why is this not working?" "What are the barriers?"

The alternative is appreciative inquiry:
- What is working well?
- How can we develop more of this?
- What do you think made it work on that occasion?
- What are the enablers of this?

Most people, whether asking, or answering, appreciative questions, are surprised at how energising it is to have conversations about what works when they or the team are operating at their best. What differentiates

Appreciative Inquiry from wishful thinking and general optimism is that it focuses on exploring *real* examples of positive events in the past or present, and thoroughly and rigorously understanding what enabled them to go well. Appreciative Inquiry has been encapsulated into a five-step method known as the 5D cycle. The first phase, *definition*, involves defining the goal and the approach; the second, *discovery*, involves participants inquiring into the times when the organisation was at its best. Phase 3 is *dreaming*, when participants describe their best picture of how the future could look. The fourth phase, *design*, requires translating the dream into reality, exploring what structures, processes, behaviours will need to change; and the last step is *destiny*, during which a range of projects are taken forward.

Through systematic appreciative story gathering and storytelling come new ideas for possible actions in the present, a confidence to experiment, and a belief and energy to create a change that builds on existing strengths and practice. Difficulties and pain are acknowledged, but are not central to the conversation or amplified. However, this requires everyone, especially leaders, to be open to what emerges rather than trying to control or second guess.

Many of the GenerationQ Fellows have found that an appreciative approach, even if not following the full five-step method, has the power to shift energy and enthusiasm for quality improvement.

Do you have to pick and choose between approaches?

In this chapter, we have explored just a selection of improvement methods. Prominent alternatives such as Business Process Re-engineering, Agile and Six Sigma have been omitted, mainly because of their lack of traction in the UK health and social care system. A question that GenerationQ Fellows often ask is what to do when faced with so many different approaches out there. So faced with this, what should you do?

Sometimes, the range of quality improvement methods can seem overwhelming. But we notice that despite each approach having its devotees, there are some similarities in them, especially with those that have originated in industry.

For most of the methods discussed, the following principles broadly apply:
- There is an emphasis on "pinning down" the issue or process that we want to work on, and on knowing what is really going on now, before we change anything. Knowing the scope of the problem and

where we want to focus is key. Standardisation and process mapping, understanding demand and capacity, are all examples of this

- In a complex system, there is often the need to isolate those key factors which will have a big impact on the problem we have identified. Identifying the constraint, value stream mapping, recording patients' moments of truth all seek to do this
- The use of data (both quantitative and qualitative) is important to make sure we get an accurate picture of the current position, and to make sure that when we make an improvement it genuinely has a beneficial effect

In the experience of the GenerationQ Fellows, the important thing is to engage in small-scale experiments to begin with and to feel neither overwhelmed nor constrained. The encouragement would be to engage in what we referred to in Chapter 1 as Trojan Mice – small, fast, under the radar experiments that give you an opportunity to have a go, to learn, to experience working with an approach in a safe way out of the limelight. Paying attention to what is going on in your context may help guide your choices. Has your organisation tried one of these approaches before? Was it successful? If not, was the reputation of the approach tarnished? If so, that might be enough to consider adopting a different approach, or at least being careful about how you brand what you do.

Understanding the particular challenges, and indeed opportunities, in your local context can also be a helpful guide. Some examples might be:
- Are you looking for colleagues to engage in small local improvement experiments? Then the model for improvement might be a good starting point
- Are you looking to increase the efficiency and effectiveness of non-clinical administrative processes? Then waste reduction and standardisation is likely to be a sound approach
- Are you looking to influence your local culture, to engage colleagues to become more patient-focused? Then Experience Based Co-Design might be your preferred option
- Is there a sense of stuckness and gloom? Then Appreciative Inquiry might help shift the mood and energy.

Wherever you start, you will probably be able to bring in principles from outside of your chosen approach, should you choose. For instance, as part of a Plan-Do-Study-Act cycle you might incorporate built-in quality principles into your improvement work. Further down the line, you might even choose to explicitly blend methods, as has been done by organisations applying Lean-Six Sigma. Whatever route you choose, you need to build in opportunities to reflect on what's gone right, what's gone wrong, opportunities to learn, opportunities to adjust your approach.

Summary

In this chapter, we have looked at five of the main methods and approaches to improve the quality of care for patients and service users. In giving this high-level tour, we have drawn attention to some of the underlying principles of these methods, and offered some examples of how they have been used in health care settings.

However, in our work with the Fellows, we have learned that this is only part of the picture. Being an expert in Lean or TOC may help lead improvement, but more is required alongside that technical understanding. In the chapter which follows, we consider other areas which a leader of quality improvement may need to address.

CHAPTER 3

Beyond the Toolkit

The proposition so far

In the previous chapters, we have described what we mean by quality, explored why improvement can be challenging and laid out the toolkit of methods which can be used to improve quality. Despite there being increased awareness of the need to improve, despite leaders generally being intelligent (sometimes brilliant), despite there being an increasing amount of writing and support around improvement methods, there are still relatively few examples of where it all goes to plan. We believe that more is needed than just good intentions and technical expertise. In this chapter, we turn to the key proposition of the book, that the toolkit is necessary and yet not sufficient, and we address the question of "What lies beyond?"

Our experience of working with health and social care leaders is that they *do* need a toolkit, or at least a good enough working knowledge of methods, which enables them to choose and commission appropriately. A method, an approach, an orientation can serve many purposes. It gives a way in, a starting point for the improvement effort. It offers a mental framework for those involved. Seeing patient pathways as a process with value- and non-value-adding steps can be a helpful piece of framing which enables people to take collective action. It offers a way of working to make those improvements, such as identifying the bottleneck or eliminating waste or discovering what we are already doing well and getting more of it.

However, to raise the tool to the status of the one truth, which will solve all ills, is to dangerously underestimate the complexity of the leadership task.

This is not uncommon, though. Sometimes quality teams seem to form almost a priesthood, with those closest to the inner sanctum being most versed in the tools and techniques of the particular method. They can also have their own language, which can alienate others who are keen to participate in improvement efforts, and, of course, every problem is the proverbial nail when solely seen from the perspective of the hammer. So, if the toolkit is necessary but not sufficient, what else is needed? If there is no single, straightforward, linear answer as to how to improve health and social care, what does lie beyond the toolkit?

The stories that follow in the rest of the book show that none of our contributors took the same path, because their individual contexts and local cultures were different. They each leaned heavily on the toolkit but did not use the same tools, or, if they did, they used them in different ways. What they do have in common, however, is that they draw on a range of skills and knowledge that can be loosely grouped around four areas, which we call the *four leadership domains*. It is this which we believe describes the territory beyond the toolkit.

The four leadership domains

Often when leadership developers think about the skills and knowledge that leaders require, they follow a well-worn path of creating a model of the ideal leader which is then translated into a series of competencies, areas in which a leader must excel to be successful. This framework and set of competencies may then be used to guide decisions about recruitment, development, promotion and remuneration. We deliberately sought to avoid this kind of prescriptive approach in our work[*]. Firstly, in our view, there is already enough pressure on leaders, like yourself, without being given an idealised, identikit picture of how you should be. Competency frameworks may be intended to inform and inspire, but often make people feel inadequate and never good enough. As one of the Fellows says:

> *How many more times am I going to be told that I am still not good enough, that I still have weaknesses that I need to address before I can be objectively recognised for doing the job that I am already doing. It is so de-moralising and de-motivating and fuels self-doubt. I have to keep on looking deep inside myself to remind myself why I bother.*

---

[*] For a full explanation of the approach to leadership development adopted for the design and delivery of GenerationQ, see Wiggins, L. and Smallwood, J. (2018, tbd). An OD Approach to Leadership Development: Questions and Consequences. *Journal of Management Development*

Secondly, in a world where issues are complex and with no simple answers, it would seem wholly incongruent for us to take an expert position and tell the senior leaders attending GenerationQ, or you the reader, how you should all be, by claiming the answer lies in following particular competencies.

Instead, we offer a much looser structure – that of four leadership domains which comprise contextual, technical, relational and personal leadership. These describe different areas of theory, research, knowledge, skill and awareness that are likely to be useful (Figure 3.1). They are intended to provide leaders, such as yourself, with a helpful framework to identify what is useful for you personally in your own context, recognising the uniqueness of both you as an individual and the shifting nature of your context. Learning to make choices about what is important and relevant for yourself, and learning to live with, and accept, some of the uncertainties and ambiguities seem to us to be part of what is essential for leading well in the 21st century.

Our intention in offering the four domains, and we will describe each in turn, is to be eclectic, inclusive, respectful and valuing of all four, recognising that the art of leadership requires all four to be woven together, integrated, in almost every gesture of leadership. Whilst each domain has a focus, putting the spotlight on certain aspects of leading, there is no intended hierarchy between them or intended suggestion that they can be useful apart from each other.

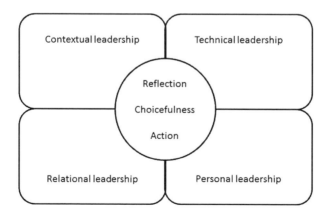

Figure 3.1: The four leadership domains

Contextual Leadership

One of the reasons we believe that quality improvement requires more than the rigorous application of a method, of a toolkit, is that context matters. In fact, context matters a great deal. It may be tempting to approach QI by simply doing "plug and play", hoping that applying an approach that worked elsewhere will deliver. However, in our experience this rarely, if ever, works because of the variation between contexts, and even within the same context over time. It is what makes leading, rather than just "doing", quality improvement an interesting but also highly sophisticated endeavour.

Difference in local culture is a major factor in contributing to variance in context, and what might work in one culture can fail dismally in another. The fact that we have a single name, "the NHS", may suggest that there is one NHS organisation and one NHS culture. However, as you are doubtless aware from your own experience, there is much variation in the way things are done and the "feel" and culture between GP surgeries and acute hospitals, between different wards and services in a single mental health Trust, between particular social enterprises and health charities. As health and social care are required to work more closely together, and in places integrate, cultural differences are often amplified. Local cultures are shaped over time as a result of different priorities and ways of doing, derived from history, geography and the personalities and preferences of past and current leaders, as well as key employees.

When the GenerationQ Fellows arrive for the first leadership forum, we thus spend some time encouraging them to explore their own context. Context can be understood as a dynamic interaction between three interlinked aspects (Jepson 2009). There is:

1. The *immediate local context* where you work. This will be affected by the personalities of others, the relationship between people, the culture that has formed over time as well as the nature of the work you and others do, and the processes that support the work, or are intended to do so. As a leader, your own perceptions and assumptions about your local context, your colleagues' readiness, willingness and ability to support improvement endeavours, will affect how confident you feel about introducing quality improvement, or may raise questions for you about what you can or can't do.

2. Your immediate local context will in turn be shaped by the *wider organisational context*. Do you work in an organisation that has been in special measures and where morale is low? Or one that has recently been merged with another so there are still competing

tribes? Have you had CEOs coming through with a regularity of revolving doors, or do you have a stable executive team where there is evident trust and a belief in the value of quality improvement? Your answers to this will shape the choices you make about how and where to undertake QI; how to start and with whom. For instance, one Fellow struggled to get QI embedded in his organisation, describing a local context of low morale and limited self-belief:

> To use a footballing analogy, we are the epitome of "mid-table mediocrity". We have a good rating from the Care Quality Commission but have poor performance against the 4-hour Accident and Emergency target. We were successful in achieving Foundation Trust status, but we remain an outlier for our rates of Hospital Acquired Infections, like clostridium difficile.

3. The third aspect of context which shapes individual organisations and systems is the *broader national context* of government, policy and regulation, of patient organisations and national and social media, as explored in Chapter 1.

These three levels of context are clearly interlinked, nested together, and influencing each other. As a leader of quality improvement, one of the skills is paying attention to them and using that awareness to make choices and decisions as to how to lead QI and how to meet the challenges described in Chapter 1.

And we mean more than this when we think about contextual leadership. We also mean being able to think about the very nature of organisations, organising and leadership in ways that help you to see new possibilities for action in your own organisational context. As we indicated in the opening chapter, one of the challenges for leaders in the health and social care context is the expectation of being in control, of having grip, of knowing what to do, of being a heroic leader. This expectation can be experienced as an overwhelming burden and comes from deeply held – often unconscious – assumptions about the very nature of organisations and leadership. In GenerationQ we offer an alternative view, informed by complexity thinking, and one where the leader is "in charge but not in control".

The invitation of the contextual leadership domain is an appeal to your head, to cognition, to thinking differently. The challenge is to probe often deeply held and unexamined assumptions about "the way things are" and how you as a leader "should" be. This can be unsettling but can also lead to liberating ways of seeing, so that you can take action from a broader behavioural repertoire. (More on this in Appendix 1: *Unpacking our mental models about organisations and leadership*.)

Technical Leadership

Technical leadership is the domain of using the toolkit wisely, deploying it thoughtfully. It is, in our view, essential for a leader in quality improvement to have some technical understanding. We say *some* technical understanding because, of all the domains, this is probably the one where it is easiest to bring in support and help, or to quickly update your knowledge and understanding through accessing widely available information. However, as a leader of quality improvement you must know enough to have credibility in the eyes of those who need to follow you, to have sufficient self-confidence and to be able to choose the most appropriate methods, and where appropriate to commission well.

The technical domain also goes beyond the methods explored in Chapter 2. It is helpful for a leader to be able to converse confidently around data, what constitutes evidence, and the use of metrics. In the quantitative data area, a basic understanding of what constitutes real change versus normal, natural fluctuations is invaluable, and can prevent knee-jerk decisions made on the basis of misunderstanding what is a genuine trend versus common cause variation. Familiarity with quantitative data can also help build credibility with clinicians, who are often trained in the scientific method and need hard data to be convinced.

The use of qualitative data, and especially patient stories, is also a powerful way of bringing alive the need for improvement, or to illustrate the impact of certain changes. Patient stories are a reminder that much of our human experience, our feelings and emotions, cannot be reduced to methods, data and measurement. Learning to appreciate the unmeasurable is also an important part of the technical domain.

Depending upon your own development and experience, a possible challenge for you within this domain might be recognising when you need to relinquish some of your desire to *know* and to be expert, particularly if this has served you well, as a clinician maybe, before progressing into taking up leadership roles.

In a leadership role, more often what is required is knowing enough to ask good questions, and to be able to delegate or commission effectively without needing to be the technical expert yourself. Leaders who are unable to do this often stifle their own ability to lead, causing paralysis and even stuckness (Watzlawick et al 1974) in their part of the organisation. Learning to be comfortable with "good enough" knowledge can be unsettling. It requires allowing others to hold that space rather than using your own expert knowledge to dominate others, to exercise power over them. It also requires letting go of the certainty that often appears to reside with the assumption of having a toolkit. While much of the technical domain is thus cognitive, being able to notice the pull towards the certainty offered by expertise and technical specialism in this domain is highly personal and emotional. Learning to lead without deep expertise can evoke the need to work with, and confront, a sense of imposter syndrome (Clance and Imes 1978), often requiring significant support. This experience will be brought to life in several of the stories.

Relational Leadership

Organisations are, by definition, social undertakings. An organisation is an attempt to bring together groups of people in ways which will enable them to work together efficiently and effectively to achieve a common purpose and goal. This domain thus encourages leaders to pay attention to, and develop, good relationships at work.

Working relationally requires a great deal of skill and takes practice. Too often, it is dismissed as "the soft stuff" of leadership, which we interpret as a defensive response because it is probably the hardest aspect of leadership. Relational leadership means being able to have genuine dialogue and honest conversations rather than debate and point scoring, or avoidance of difficult issues. Patricia Shaw (2002), one of the writers we ask the Fellows to read, talks of change happening one conversation at a time. Reframing meetings as conversations, even if it is just in your own head, immediately makes them more human, more relational, less formal. Creating the conditions for conversations, where there is reciprocity with an intention to both listen and understand, requires paying attention to what may be small things but which can have significant impact, such as where to meet, the physical set-up of a room and how a meeting starts. It is a reminder too of the importance of asking others, of inquiry, or what Heron (2009) calls "pull" gestures, rather than "push" gestures where we take charge and tell and advocate from our perspective, which can easily lead to stuck patterns of interaction and frustration.

Learning how to engage well with power and navigate organisational politics with skill are also recurring themes in the Fellows' stories. At the beginning of the programme, many talk of relying on either the power that comes with the job title and their place in the organisational or professional hierarchy, which is known as positional power, or their technical expertise, which is known as expert power. However, we encourage viewing power in a much more fluid and dynamic way, as something which can be grown and developed and exists within relationships rather than as an individual possession. Instead of talking about "power over" others, which sits with the heroic leadership model, we encourage talk of "power with", the synergy which emerges through building engagement and collaboration with others, and "power within", the self-awareness, confidence and self-acceptance that comes with recognising that, as a leader, you cannot control all that happens and you have your own strengths and limitations.

We see politics as neutral and a recognition of the fact that in any organisation there will be different interests at play. In health and social care organisations and systems, there are multiple stakeholders. This is why we identified one of the six challenges of leading quality improvement in Chapter 1, as "brokering sufficient stakeholder participation and agreement". There are no simple answers, but here are some principles the Fellows have found helpful. One is to make it your business to try and see the world from the perspective of other stakeholders in the system. What are the pressures on them? Why might they be acting like that? Are you at risk of making assumptions based on history, or seeing them as a "generalised other" rather than a specific individual? For instance, it is easy to dismiss a whole group of people with wide sweeping generalisations: "Oh well, doctors always say ....."; "Nurses will never do....". If in doubt, go and have an inquiry conversation and explore what is really important to them. This leads to another helpful concept – the difference between front stage and back stage conversations (Buchanan and Boddy 1992). Front stage meetings are those formal ones which often follow a set pattern, where there is a great deal of positional power present and the alliances may not be overt or visible. Back stage conversations are those where you can have a more informal dialogue to float an idea past someone, to build connection and relationship, to get a sense of their interest or objections without either you or them feeling that your answers need to be filtered by what others might say or think.

Other challenges we mentioned in Chapter 1 included "leading others in complex change" and "making informed choices about when and how to act". Here some of the skills include knowing how much to come up with your own ideas, and how much to encourage others and work with what emerges. It means understanding what goes on in groups and teams and knowing how to help them to work at their best. It involves understanding some of the natural human reaction to change, including the emotions that are inevitably evoked, and learning how to help people make changes for themselves. It means understanding aspects of human psychology to limit anxiety so that people feel comfortable enough to offer their best. It certainly involves knowing how, and when, to run a meeting which achieves something and isn't just a ritualistic gathering which clutters up the day. It means understanding why people disagree and why there is conflict, and having some strategies to deal with these kinds of situations.

The list of skills may well sound daunting. The upside of relational leadership, however, is that just small shifts in your behaviour can bring about significant, profound and transformational change – albeit unpredictable. Transformation doesn't have to be big or grand. It can be a different move or gesture on your part, an act of offering feedback, an act of staying quiet and listening well. You will read a lot about the impact of seemingly small shifts of behaviour in the stories, and as one Fellow recounts:

> *I tentatively broached the nursing team again. Previous encounters had not gone well. Initially I had tried to passionately offer them my vision for a new pathway. When this didn't work I tried to sell the benefits. And then, when this again didn't work I labelled the team as negative and was left sitting with my own frustration! This time I elected to try out a more relational leadership style, including more active listening. I spoke less and, rather than being defensive, I consciously demonstrated vulnerability by acknowledging uncertainties. Once I sensed some engagement I attempted to use "pull" rather than "push" questions. A pivotal point came when I named that I sensed there were mixed feelings which hadn't previously been acknowledged. The team begun to focus their comments on the positives and appeared to be more enthusiastic about the pathway, so I followed this up by asking how they saw it (the pathway) developing. By this point they were now offering their concerns, ideas and suggested changes. I became a surprisingly willing bystander as they self-organised roles in development, implementation and audit of the new pathway. I was astounded at how much difference these seemingly small changes in my gestures had made. Perhaps unsurprisingly, although I had not predicted it, much of their true concern focused on having potentially difficult discussions over the telephone. What was interesting for me was that acknowledging this was enough for them, it did not need to be "solved", particularly not by me.*

Many theories appertaining to relational leadership are described in *Relational Change: the art and practice of changing organizations* by Wiggins and Hunter (2016). Brief overviews of Transactional Analysis (Berne 1967; Lapworth and Sills 2011), Push and Pull (Heron 2009) and Dialogue (Isaacs 1999) are also included in Appendix 2: *Relational Dynamics*.

Personal Leadership

You, as an individual, will bring much to the role of leading quality improvement. You will bring your history, your experience, your relationships and your knowledge. It is also helpful for you to be aware of your strengths, your personal patterns, your biases, your impact upon others and your blind spots. Knowing these in yourself can help you spot them in other people, and help you choose the appropriate gesture to make, at a given point.

The personal domain is the area where most competency-based leadership development programmes tend to focus (Pedler et al 2004). It is also an area where psychometrics, such as MBTI, provide labels and insights into the self and how individuals differ from each other. In our experience on GenerationQ, leading requires going beyond psychometrics into more personal psychology to enhance self-awareness and self-acceptance. This is because engaging others in change can involve uncertainty and anxiety, inviting others to project their fears or anger onto the leader. This is why another of the six challenges we identify for leading quality improvement is "sustaining self and others". So leaders need to be aware enough of their own patterns, defences and triggers to be able to recognise what is their "stuff" and what is other people's. This is essential for staying psychologically safe and grounded, for connecting with others and for developing personal resilience.

As with the relational leadership domain, there is a wide range of interesting theories and ideas that support awareness and understanding of personal leadership. We consider two here that are mentioned in many of the Fellows' stories later in the book: personal drivers (Kahler and Capers 1974) and the role and place for vulnerability (Brown 2012; Brown 2010).

On GenerationQ, many of the Fellows say that the notion of personal drivers has helped them understand their own behaviour patterns, as well as those of other people. Personal drivers are formed in childhood. As children we create a narrative or "life script" based largely on the encouragements and reprimands that we receive from parents and early care givers. These social messages about what is expected of us continue to exert a powerful influence on us as adults. There are five drivers: Please People, Be Perfect, Be Strong, Hurry Up and Try Hard. We often have one or two which dominate and these can be sources of real strength. However, overplayed or overused as a default way of responding to situations, they can lead us to tripping ourselves up or getting enmeshed in stuck patterns. Once you know your own drivers, you can make sense of a particular situation that made you frustrated; you can catch yourself in the moment when you experience a strong emotion, and understand why that might be; and you can consider choicefully what moves to make next, rather than acting out of habit. There is more detail on personal drivers and a questionnaire in Appendix 3 if you wish to learn more about your own drivers and how they might play out in your own leadership.

Brené Brown (2012) explores the role of vulnerability and leadership. Based on her extensive research, she proposes that true strength lies in our ability to acknowledge our need for others, rather than trying to be the heroic leader who tries to do everything single-handed. It takes real courage to accept that we do not have all the answers, but if we are able to show some vulnerability, to acknowledge what or when we don't know, to admit that we too have made mistakes, we allow others to see us as real human beings. This enables a different kind of connection and more trusting relationships at work. Of course, sometimes in the culture of health care there are those who might see vulnerability as a weakness which should be hidden and suppressed. Here too there are therefore choices to be made as a leader – when is it useful to share vulnerability and when not?

Here one of the Fellows, who is a medical director, shares his reflections on what others may see as a paradox between power and vulnerability, but he sees as a strength:

> *I was attending an Integration Board Development day with health and social care. This was about setting our strategy for the next five years. It went on for a long time and I said little … until the end. I had been holding a thought and finally articulated it; it was around changing our approach to service users … I used two personal stories, one I got wrong, one I got right, to strengthen my argument and was conscious of holding some silences and demonstrating emotion without offering any form of apology. At the end there was silence then a new conversation started, building on my comments and, ultimately, leading to a new direction. I could feel the difference in me both during and after that monologue. I was aware that I was making myself vulnerable but resisted any move to apologise for both that and for any discomfort in the room. It felt good. It felt powerful. Afterwards a colleague from Social Work approached me and thanked me for articulating what he felt was key to changing the tone and direction of the conversation which he felt had been essential to creating the potential for a new culture.*

Developing a "third eye"

At the beginning of this chapter we emphasised the importance of all four domains, of holding them together in every act of leadership. As highlighted in Figure 3.1, central to this is the ability to *integrate*, *reflect* and make a conscious *choice* about how to act in the moment, and often how to *experiment* in acting differently. We choose to call this ability developing your third eye. This is closely akin to ideas of developing a reflective practice, and continuous learning from experience.

Imagine we could now magically give you an invisible extra eye, which some may visualise as a sophisticated parking mirror that allows you to see where you are in relation to others. Others talk about the third eye as if it were on a long arm that can swivel round so that you can look at yourself from a new angle. Some enjoy becoming creative and envisage an eye on a wiggly antenna like an alien in a children's book. Visualisations aside, the key concept here is looking at yourself and your situation from different perspectives. The third eye gives you two new abilities. The first is the ability to recognise that in every situation, especially those where you are leading, you see the world through the filter of your own assumptions and metaphors. Yet every situation can be seen from a range of different perspectives, and your perspective – and importantly your awareness of your perspective – is crucial in determining what you do and how you act. The encouragement here is to remember your view is just one perspective and to inquire into others.

The second ability is to see yourself in the moment, to observe yourself as if from the outside, to reflect and then make a conscious choice about how to act rather than being on automatic pilot. Heifetz (2002) describes this as getting off the dance floor to observe yourself from the balcony. Two Fellows comment on how they experienced learning to reflect and develop their third eye:

> Being asked to reflect more was hard at first, but I am really seeing things differently now. I can choose how to react rather than running on auto-pilot.

> It's all very well reflecting on my perspectives before or after the event. The harder thing seems to be to be able to pause in the moment and catch myself before I do something without consideration.

Reflecting in this way means more than simply remembering or musing or ruminating. Reflection means examining your own actions and their consequences, with the purpose of seeing what it can teach you. David Kolb (1984) created a model for adult learning which we often use on the GenerationQ programme and which illustrates how reflective practice might work.

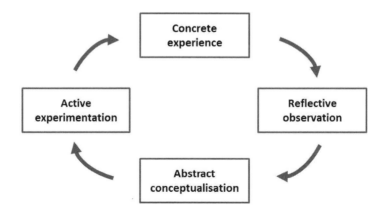

Figure 3.2. Source: David Kolb, Experiential Learning (1984)

Let us take an imaginary example to help bring this to life. Imagine you are leading a piece of quality improvement work and are full of enthusiasm. One day you are meeting with your colleagues. All seems to be going well as you explain why this is so exciting and why you are so passionate about it, and how it will really change the patient experience, and then there is a reaction from one of the people at the meeting. "It won't work here," she says, and goes on to explain in negative terms how this has been tried before and is now ridiculed by staff.

You are deflated and depressed. Perhaps you should stop now. Perhaps you are not inspirational enough as a leader, perhaps you don't have the charisma required to pull this off.

Then you remember that everything has something to teach us, and you decide to reflect. You follow the Kolb Cycle of thinking about the *Concrete Experience*, what happened, who was there, how was the room laid out, what was the temperature. You move to *Reflective Observation*, how did you feel, who was saying what, what might he have been thinking, what was really going on? You use *Abstract Conceptualisation* to try to make sense of this experience. Perhaps you were speaking too much and not listening. Perhaps the harder you push, the more others feel the need to counteract your excessive enthusiasm. Perhaps the negative colleague was asking for reassurance and support. You might turn to relevant theory to help you make sense or to surface assumptions you might be holding. You complete the cycle by moving to *Active Experimentation*: What could you try next? What might your reflections have taught you and how will you be different next time?

By making reflection a habit, you give yourself a chance of finding different ways through the complexities of your situation. To encourage the Fellows in this, we suggest they write their reflections in a journal. Joining an action learning set, or engaging a coach also helps because this provides the discipline of meetings with others to support your reflection. The additional benefits of reflection in the moment are that you give yourself a range of options rather than auto-pilot. You also give yourself hope. You are not condemned to continue the same strategies and approaches you have always used. You can become a dynamic and effective leader, adapting to changing circumstances as you go, growing and developing as you learn from your experience. You can do more than survive the challenges of leading QI. You can thrive.

Summary

In this chapter, we have introduced the four domains of contextual, technical, relational and personal leadership. Our intention is to give some light structure to different areas of theory, research, knowledge, skill and awareness that are likely to be useful to you as a leader of quality improvement. This is what lies beyond the toolkit. To illustrate how individual leaders have drawn on these domains, as they address the practical challenges of quality improvement in their own context, we turn now to the stories.

As we mentioned in the introduction, the stories are written by the Fellows themselves, and they provide a rarely heard account of what it is like to lead in practice, "warts and all". Each story represents the perspective of one individual. They each share their experience of what actually happened when they were making moves to change things for the better in their workplace. As such, the stories represent their truth, their learning, their inner dialogue about what they thought and felt, what they did and why. And, as we will all recognise, whenever any of us recount what happened at work our accounts are always partial, because we choose what to share, what to leave out. The Fellows' stories are therefore not attempting to represent "the truth" or a definitive answer to "what actually happened". Their intention is to tell their story to be helpful to others who may be in similar situations. It is not to create an objective, scientific account.

A few other observations: care has been taken to disguise the identity of the organisations and individuals within each story, to avoid any risk of unintentionally offending others. As the stories are written by the Fellows themselves, the writing styles vary, reflecting their different voices.

Experimenting
Finding fertile ground

This first section of stories from the Fellows is united by the theme of beginning, of starting something. The contributors, driven by a desire or the necessity to improve the quality of health care, all faced the same fundamental questions – how and where to begin? Every journey must begin with a single step, said Lao Tzu, and the same is true here; without beginning there is no possibility of anything happening.

But there is more than just the theme of beginning in these stories. There is also a sense of tentativeness – a recognition that beginning something, making an initial move, brings with it a sense of risk. The Fellows are asking people to change something, change the process, change their behaviour, and are aware that they may not want to, they may reject these initial moves.

On the GenerationQ programme, we discuss and explore some of our thinking around complexity, and how, in organisational life, the complexity of the interactions between individuals with free will means that a leader cannot predict, or ever fully control, what will happen when she makes this kind of move or gesture, as we call it (for more explanation of this see Appendix 1). The "meaning" of the gesture may not be what the leader intended, in that its meaning lies in how the gesture is interpreted. If a leader cannot predict and cannot control what is going to happen, then these beginnings will always be somewhat tentative, and in these stories the Fellows learn that they must pay attention to how the gestures land, and adjust their subsequent behaviour accordingly. We have chosen to call this "experimenting".

Framing these actions as experimenting in this way is, we believe, very useful in helping leaders to begin the process of quality improvement. The central point about this kind of experiment is that it doesn't matter if it works in the way it is intended or not. Either way, something has begun and some valuable information about what works is now available, and next steps can be shaped accordingly.

But we are not advocating that leaders simply begin in any way and in any place. What these stories also have in common is the choice of a context and an approach where there is a chance that the experiment will lead to some improvement. In some cases, the choice is thrust upon them, but still requires the Fellow to think about which approach will really get to the bottom of the issue and result in sustainable improvement. A quote from one of our stories says this better than we can: "It's not that you can control what will happen but you are tilling the soil, preparing the earth for seeds that will hopefully germinate."

There are four stories in this section, each offering insight into the early stages of improving quality in health care:
- The first, *Shouting at a Flower Doesn't Make It Grow*, describes an improvement born out of a crisis. Performance in a particular department is causing great concern, and much blame is being passed around. Rather than colluding with these accusations, our contributor recognised that "a different approach was needed", an experiment which moved away from allocating blame, or treating the symptoms, to a brave gesture to take a more fundamental improvement approach.
- The second, *Lessening the Roar*, describes a clinician exploring how to get improvement to stick in different departments. He finds that by inquiring more and telling less, staff will often own the change themselves.
- The third, *Getting Out of the Way*, explores attempts to get positive engagement in a team, and examines how "huddles" can be improved when the leader pays attention to relationships and offers empathy.
- The fourth, *Moving through Treacle, Discovering Pearls*, tells of a clinician's attempt to introduce Theory of Constraints to their division, with some contrasting results; one area enthusiastically adopts the approach whilst other colleagues are less keen.

These four stories illustrate the fascinating interplay between the theories of improvement (the "toolkit") and the reality of using them in patient care. They offer us lessons, sometimes hard learned, about the dangers of heroically mounting a white horse and charging into the fray, certain that the approach we have is going to revolutionise the service. Of course, changing things and working with others turns out to be much messier and much less clear cut than our contributors thought. The situation requires them to hold their toolkit lightly, to recognise that it is not a cure-all, to experiment, and to work hard on relationships and how others are seeing the situation.

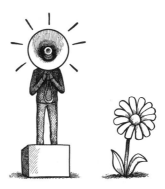

CHAPTER **4**

Shouting at a Flower Doesn't Make It Grow

We are falling over as a Trust. Performance is going down the pan and if we don't get this sorted most of us aren't going to have jobs. So you need to get things fixed and they need fixing now. I know you can deliver because you sort things... Focus on Ophthalmology – get in there, sort them out... They are messing around and I'm sick of them. Change the behaviours. Change the numbers. Understand?

I paraphrase slightly since the conversation was littered with expletives. The CEO was alternating between jabbing his forefinger in the air and punching his fist into his hand. I expect he was feeling under pressure himself. He was certainly now dumping the angst on me. I was also told I would need to get a clinical lead to work with, someone who, in his words, "needs to be prepared to do some kicking".

Some weeks later, I was summoned back: "Come on then, how many of this lot am I going to have to sack to turn this round?" (CEO)

My heart sank. At my interview the CEO had been part of the panel, and I had talked at length about my ambition to be part of what he had described as "embedding continuous improvement at every level within the organisation". This was the same person now telling me to "Just sort the performance. You can do your improvement stuff once we are back on track and off the radar".

In my recently appointed role as Divisional Director, I had responsibility across a broad range of surgical, critical care, diagnostic and outpatient specialties. Within this was Ophthalmology, a large specialty that nationwide accounts for 10 percent of all outpatient appointments. It is an area of rapidly increasing demand with an ever-growing list of "planned" patients needing ongoing monitoring and treatment, as well as new patients. It's also an area of astonishing innovation where new treatments and interventions are improving and saving vision. Timeliness is often vital to avoid serious deterioration, or even loss of sight. I hadn't been long in the role when we discovered a group of patients waiting for treatment who had been "lost to follow-up". Tragically we were later to find that two of them had already suffered significant and irreversible deterioration in their sight as a result of this delay.

Ophthalmology in this hospital was a department with a long history of such problems, and everyone seemed exhausted and battle weary. The admin staff were demoralised, sickness rates were high, and it wasn't unusual for someone to be in tears. The clinical lead, Gavin, an experienced Ophthalmologist, was a feisty, animated man. He was clinically excellent, the doctor that others always recommended if you wanted any of your own family treating or an opinion sought. I trusted what he said, but often felt like I was walking on eggshells around him. You had to catch him at the right time to ask him a question, or talk about putting on extra lists. If not, he could blast you with a tirade of exasperation about the Trust, the management or the Chief Executive. He could alternate between shouting in frustration and being highly charming. I had to keep reminding myself that he cared deeply about the service, and that these outbursts came from a place of sheer frustration and stress, but it felt uncomfortable tolerating it and not challenging him.

Performance was "managed" in the Trust at a weekly performance meeting. Amanda, the COO and my line manager, told me that the intense external scrutiny of Trust performance had resulted in the exec team deciding to lead the meetings themselves. "It's to show everyone we have grip on what's going on in the organisation," she told me. Every Wednesday at 9am we would file into the Executive Meeting Room, arranging ourselves around the long oval table. We would all flick through sheets of paper or check our emails, hoping the answer to our final query had dropped into our inbox before the spotlight was on us. It was hushed, formal and tense as the focus moved from person to person. The relief when you were off the hook and had survived your few minutes of questioning; the humiliation when your answer was deemed inadequate. From some colleagues, sympathetic looks or supportive smiles; from others smirks or rolling of eyes. One time, before we had filed in, a colleague joked about who was going to wear the bullseye target tabard that day. I'm sure I wasn't the only one asking, why are we doing this? We were grown adults but we were being treated like naughty children by critical and continuously disappointed parents. No, that feels too mild. It felt more like the Spanish Inquisition. It was a meeting that symbolised a culture of manic, hamster-wheel-like activity where being seen to be scurrying around was what seemed to be valued. The culture was so all pervasive it felt impossible to stand up and say stop, hang on, what are we all doing here?

As anxiety levels for both us and the exec team increased, it felt as though getting through the meetings became more important than actually finding solutions or real improvements. I asked one of the managers, who had been in the organisation for some time, how she felt and was taken aback by her reply:

"It's like tiptoeing through a dark wood with all these eyes staring at you, waiting to trip you up, catch you out or stab you in the back. I certainly wouldn't ask any of them for help."

Against this backdrop, the extent of what was happening in Ophthalmology began to emerge. A new performance monitoring system had recently been introduced as part of upgrading and modernising our processes, and this was starting to provide much more clarity and depth on all our waiting lists, not just our 18 week pathways. At the same time changes in the information being requested by commissioners was leading to greater interrogation of the data. We began to uncover the extent of the backlog of patients waiting for treatment who had previously been "hidden", not reported in the waiting time data, since they were planned and therefore no longer on an 18 week pathway. I needed to know more, to get clarity on the true position, but the more I looked and asked questions and gathered data, the more confusing and contradictory was the picture that emerged. Analysts, performance teams, commissioners and the Ophthalmology Department all held different versions of the truth, but all agreed that the number of patients waiting was large, growing and seemingly out of control. Finding an agreed and consistent way of collecting reliable data, that everyone believed in, was going to have to be a priority. There were also multiple explanations offered of whose "fault" it was that our lists were growing and ever changing, and where the solution lay.

"There's not enough capacity."

"It's the data."

"It's the lack of data."

"The Trust won't fund the right number of doctors."

"We haven't got enough nurses to staff the procedure lists."

"We don't get given the correct information to book the patients."

"There's huge growth in demand and we can't keep up."

"We don't get given the right notice to cancel the lists."

"We don't know how to work out who to book."

"You'll have to ask Sue / Neil / Sandy – they devised their own system, separate from the Trust process, and seemed to stay on top of things."

I knew from experience that there were probably grains of truth in all these comments. Complex problems like this rarely have a single answer, much as many of us, including me, might yearn for it!

I was meeting Amanda, my line manager, for our weekly one to one. Walking along the executive corridor to her office, I bumped into the CEO.

"Haven't you got Ophthalmology sorted yet? Thought you said at interview that you'd done an improvement course, so what's taking the time? You just need to tell them what to do." I stood there trying to work out what to say, but he turned on his heel and left.

Amanda, the COO, was, like me, relatively new in post, having moved into the Trust from a regional role. She hadn't worked before at a senior level in operational management and was leaking anxiety, twisting her wedding ring round and round her finger. Before the meeting, I'd been thinking about what to say to Amanda – I knew that we needed to take some action urgently but was also aware that giving false certainty wasn't going to be helpful either. On the GenerationQ programme I'd learned how it feels to be a "torn middle" caught between those above you, the "tops", putting on pressure, clamouring for an answer and a solution, and those below you in the system, the "bottoms", needing time and air cover to pause in the hectic activity of their work to explore and experiment with different ways of doing things.

Amanda looked deeply uncomfortable when I said I couldn't give her the certainty of an immediate solution. Her lips tightened and I could see blotches appearing on her neck and face.

"Look, I shouldn't need to tell you there's no place for not knowing right now. You need to be seen to be doing something, and quickly," she said.

Here was further confirmation of what I had already been noticing about the culture here: that what you looked as though you were doing was often, at least in the short term, deemed as important as what you were *actually* doing.

There was a pause...and then she skewered me with one of those throw away comments that hurt and undermine.

"Of course, Kelly, the last service manager they had in there, was really committed to improving things. She had a real grasp of the situation and was there every night, even at the weekend sometimes, going through all the patient cards. She knew every patient who was waiting, or at least was on the lists."

I could feel my heart racing at this, and forced myself to breathe slowly. The blame game in action. I knew getting cross wouldn't be helpful. I took a long, steadying sip of coffee. It was tepid. I so resented the unfairness of being on the receiving end of this, and another bit of me knew that Amanda was also passing on the pressure and finger pointing from the CEO, who was himself experiencing it from the regulator. Both of them were "torn middles" with the regulator as their "top". Being able to draw on the theory helped me stay calm in the moment by making sense of what was happening; seeing us all as part of a system under pressure rather than "bad" individuals.

Even though I didn't know what the answer was, I was absolutely certain that me working all night, or asking someone else to do so, was not the solution. Everyone in the department said the constant fire-fighting had been going on for as long as anyone could remember.

A few days later I met up with my GenerationQ action learning set and shared the real mix of emotions I was experiencing. I was really cross. I felt tricked into joining and working in the Trust because they had said they were interested in creating an open and honest culture, supporting staff and embedding improvement, when the reality felt so different. I felt embarrassed that I didn't know the answers in the onslaught of the expectations that I should. Having participated on GenerationQ, a programme all about leadership of improvement, the critical voice in my own head was adding to the pressure – perhaps I should know what to do? I felt frustrated that I was being told to play the game of making it look like we were doing something to solve the problem, rather than actually working through what we needed. I felt worried that the clinicians would just dig their heels in and refuse to help. Gavin, the clinical lead had already told me last time I asked about some additional capacity, "Don't think we are going to do loads of extra lists just to save 'their' jobs", and, underpinning it all, I think I was actually quite frightened. Frightened of the consequences for all those patients left waiting, frightened of failing, of not being to fix it and of falling flat on my face in a new job in front of everyone.

My default reaction was to think that I needed to sort this out, and sorting it meant getting in there and doing it myself. People were looking to me for the answer, and as the leader I should know what to do – and get on and do it. This was driven in part by the dominant organisational culture to reward the "heroic leader" who saves the day (or looks like they have), but I think there was more to it than that. On GenerationQ, I'd learned about personal drivers, unconscious internal pressures which are based on the messages we are given when we are young about what is expected of us and what is rewarded. I have a firmly embedded Be Strong driver so I am calm under pressure, good at sorting problems and making things happen, with a reputation for self-sufficiency, reliability, and delivery (Lapworth and Sills, 2011) (See Appendix 3). I am a survivor, and this has served me well through some really tough times, both inside and outside of work. A shadow side of this driver is a fear of rejection and exposing vulnerability, so asking for help, and saying "I don't know" really goes against the grain. With this knowledge of my own personal leadership patterns, I knew that going in and trying to single-handedly sort it out would mean I would take on all the responsibility for finding a solution; everyone else would feel disempowered; there would be no ownership, and I would in effect be managing or trying to be a lone hero and do it all myself.

There's a link here with one of the questions I, and others, often grappled with on GenerationQ. What does it actually mean to *lead* improvement as opposed to do it? How much expertise in different improvement methodologies is required of me to personally lead and implement the improvement project in Ophthalmology? Or does my leadership role as Director require a different set of skills and knowledge, creating the conditions for others to be "doing the doing"?

Asking for help

The first people I spoke to about some help were the Trust service improvement team, but the work was outside their annual plan. They gave me their QI Users' Guide but I knew enough about different improvement methodologies to know we required a really detailed look at data, systems and processes; this might not fit the simplicity of the PDSA plan set out in their paperwork, and the staff working in the Ophthalmology department would need to be involved. I was managing a range of services so I knew I couldn't devote all my time to Ophthalmology, and I wasn't sure I had sufficient knowledge of the right methodologies to use in detail to lead and implement this type of work. I decided I needed to bring in some intensive technical expertise, but knew that it also needed to be someone who had the relational skills to work with staff, and someone whom I could trust.

Mel and I had worked together in my previous Trust and I thought she would be ideal. She was from Manchester, slightly built, with long ginger hair that she wore swept up into a bun, with locks always escaping. She worked hard and had the ability to get on with everyone, treating everyone the same whatever their level in the hierarchy. If you asked her what she enjoyed about her job, her standard reply was "I love making organisational life a little less bonkers and a bit more organised".

I needed to use all my relational skills to get colleagues to agree to Mel joining. There were lots of back stage conversations which to be honest felt a bit annoying, as I was so convinced Mel would give us the extra capacity and knowledge we needed. However, I knew that getting buy-in is part of any change and was critical to creating the conditions for Mel being successful.

"Isn't this just throwing good money after bad?" asked Amanda, the COO. I showed her the investment required to fund four months of Mel's time versus what we were paying to private providers to manage some of the backlog.

"Another consultant – really?" said Gavin, the clinical lead. "Do we really need someone else coming in who doesn't understand the service, asks loads of questions, and then tells us what to do?"

"Why don't you meet Mel and see if you could work with her?" I said to Gavin, wanting him to feel some choice in this rather than me imposing Mel on him. It was a small gesture that in hindsight had a significant impact, because it broke the pattern of him feeling "done to" by management.

So, eventually I secured the funding and commitment for four months of Mel's support.

When Mel arrived, two weeks later, it was such a relief to be working alongside someone whom I could trust and speak with openly. I now had a thought partner, as an equal, with whom to mull over what we were learning, what themes were emerging, the choice of next steps to take. I felt less alone. I felt better able to notice the dominant culture and to begin to create a different local context where there was time to think.

On Mel's first day, we walked up to the department together so I could introduce her to the booking team in the administration office. As we stood in the doorway, I noticed Mel's eyes darting around, taking it all in as she tucked an escaped lock of hair behind her ear.

The office is long, narrow and stuffy, lit by a harsh strip light. Teetering piles of documents are scattered around with barely a piece of workstation identifiable under the mass of paper, multi-coloured cards, keyboards, phones, patient notes and in-trays labelled "For vetting", "For grading". Post-its cling to monitors; white scrappy notes form makeshift titles for the piles of papers they rest upon. Boxes of envelopes and treatment packs are shoved under desks. Laminated signs on the walls have amendments on post-it notes stuck over the top of them. And still more paper is flooding in: people in blue scrubs walk down the office, leaning over to stuff another referral into already overflowing Perspex slots on the wall.

Along the narrow office are half a dozen people, mostly on the phone speaking to patients. It's September and the office is unbearably hot. Desk fans whirr away, wafting sheets of paper pinned to the boards on the walls. Mark, one of the booking clerks, rests his phone's handset on the desk and spins his chair around, his brow crinkled. Gavin, the Ophthalmology clinical lead pushes past us and homes in on Mark. "What's this woman doing on my list?" he shouts. "It doesn't take a senior to perform a routine cataract removal. A complete waste of my time." Mark stares at the green piece of paper that Gavin has thrust in his hand. "My mistake," says Mark. Gavin shakes his head and spins on his heel. As he leaves the room he turns to Mel and me and says, "Best of luck with this. You really think you can sort it out?"

We wanted to speak to Tricia, the team leader, but our conversation is staccato, punctuated by her answering calls: "Sorry, they've put you through to the wrong department." "I'm sorry you've not received your drops, I'll get some more sent out to you." We leave, conscious that we are adding to the activity and distracting the team.

Later that week, I suggest Mel and I meet the IT team who have been producing the data for the department. It is a fraught meeting, as the IT analyst explains that they have just found an extra 37 patients and they are not sure what is happening with them, or why they have suddenly appeared on the system. One of the patients appears to have waited over 20 weeks for his treatment. How can this be? I'm *so* frustrated.

"What do you mean? How can you just find another 37 patients?! Where have they come from?"

Later Mel says to me, "You know that Spanish Inquisition you were talking about, and how horrible it was? I didn't realise you were one of the interrogators!" And as soon as she said it, I realised with horror she was right. My own style was becoming impacted by the dominant culture.

This was a wake-up call for me. As a relative newcomer I had got into the habit of thinking I was sitting outside the system, looking in on it, as if I was an impartial observer, reassuring myself: "I'm not like that, its everyone else who is behaving badly"; or perhaps sometimes feeling like a victim: "It's not fair; everyone is being so unreasonable". In fact, the analyst in IT had had no involvement in the origin of the information, the clinical decision, or the way the data was entered or organised on the system, and yet here I was directing my frustration about the situation onto him. It was tough hearing Mel's comment, but she was absolutely right to draw my attention to my own behaviour in this context.

Choosing to lead

Mel worked with the booking team and created a small team of five that also included Gavin the senior clinician, the lead nurse, and Tricia the head of the admin team. Over the next two months they worked together, process mapping every step from referral to treatment, timing every action and interaction, counting and coding every patient, every procedure, every action. I met with the team weekly. In the first few meetings, I felt a bit left out of the work. It felt strange not getting into every detail; slightly risky, and certainly not what I would have done in my previous role as a manager. However, I came to see that what I was doing as the leader in the meeting was creating a thinking space, somewhere for the team to stop and pause, away from the frenetic hamster wheel of activity, to articulate what they were learning and explore things they were struggling with. My role was to ask good inquiry questions, to affirm what was going well and to coach the team around possible solutions or next steps. I was also learning enough in the meetings to be able to provide a sense of progress to the board, so that there was air cover for the team against stresses and pressures from the exec team.

Owning the data

Getting the right data and information was one of the big challenges I'd identified early on. Mel agreed. When we started the work, weekly reports were produced by the performance team in Finance, who passed them to the lead nurse, who passed them to Tricia and her admin team to inform them which patients to book. At the same time, a demand and capacity tool was being developed by the information team to help plan the number of required lists. A member of the central improvement team had been working on a separate tool to develop the improvement trajectory, required to ensure the department would hit the required targets by the end of the year. Yet none of these reports aligned with each other, and the admin team felt bombarded with conflicting information and powerless to know which ones to use as the principal source of information. There was also so little confidence in the reports that the Trust employed full time validators to go through them, correcting information entered inaccurately in the first place because they didn't tally with the clinical notes. No one in the admin team was able to access the source data for any of this, and they were passive recipients of all of this information. Solberg (1997) talks about "drowning in sea of data", and it certainly felt like that here.

The team's summary of their initial diagnostic phase was:
- 6,500 referrals in 48 different places in the office (drawers, shelves, folders, boxes, files)
- 45 percent of patient referrals put onto the system incorrectly the first time so people spend time correcting and validating the data in the system
- Multiple referral routes in from GPs, other consultants, clinical nurse specialists, planned waiting list, internal Ophthalmology clinics, neighbouring Trusts
- Constant interruptions to the admin team from staff asking them to swap patients, change lists or find information, and phone calls from patients wanting to know what was happening
- Out of date information printed out and laminated about which doctor can perform which procedure to support booking patients on the correct lists

Amanda confirmed that Ophthalmology performance was going to be discussed at the next board performance meeting. I knew that in sharing these findings I was going to be exposing our weaknesses and problems, and I wasn't yet able to also explain what the solution was, and when the performance would improve. It wasn't a message that anyone wanted to hear. Amanda, the COO, was anxious:

"You can't keep promising them you are going to sort this when you have got no improvement to show them. I think you should take some of the Ophthalmology staff in with you. The team needs to realise how serious this is, and you need to demonstrate that you are holding their feet to the fire."

I refused. The team knew the seriousness of the situation. The procession of managers through their department to chase performance, the never-ending phone calls with distressed patients hoping for their appointment, they were in no doubt about that. My role was to provide some space and protection from that to allow them to work together with Mel to develop and implement the improvements.

I presented the data. I survived.

Later that day, Mel and I went to meet the IT Director, Christine.

"We'd really like to get to a place where the operational team in Ophthalmology own their own data," said Mel with enthusiasm.

Christine was one of those "yes-but" people who seem good at finding reasons for saying no, but does so in a way that is positioned, and I think intended, as being helpful.

"You've got to be really careful there … we did that once in another Trust where I used to work. Incorrect information was given to one of our partner organisations. Operational teams don't understand these sort of sensitivities. Much safer if we hold the data as the IT department, especially given concerns about data security." No budging her.

Local data ownership was a significant issue though. I hadn't realised how disempowering the current policy was until I heard the team talk in one of our project meetings. I decided that now was the time to be 10 percent braver.

"OK, rather than fighting the current system, let's develop and test our own processes, and keep the work under the radar to give ourselves time to experiment and develop an approach that works for us," I said. "What we are doing is giving ourselves some space to try a few different things out, see what happens, and take it from there," I told them, "a few small, quick experiments that go unseen." Gavin was excited. Mark and Tricia were apprehensive. Were we allowed to do this? What if someone found out? This was asking them to work outside their comfort zone and the normal culture of just doing what you were told, but with Mel's support and skills and my reassurance they were willing to give it a go.

"I'll take responsibility; if anyone questions it just ask them to speak to me," I assured them. As it was, no one ever questioned us about these rapid cycle experiments, some might say Trojan mice experiments, and away from the direct scrutiny they tried and tested, tried and tested.

One of the most significant changes we made was to take away the preparation and maintenance of operational and performance data from the central teams and place it in the hands of the Ophthalmology admin team. They were so used to in-putting swathes of data on a daily basis and seeing it disappear into a data abyss, that storing and analysing their own data felt alien at first, then liberating. They started to talk with confidence about which patients were waiting, what demands were placed on the service, and what capacity they had with which to meet them.

Once they were able to develop their daily work flow themselves, working with a dataset that they knew was reliable and up to date as they were producing it direct from patient records, they could also talk with confidence to patients about the waiting position. The waits were still long, but at least they were now known.

Slowly, over the next two months, the detailed and systematic work that the team was undertaking with Mel's supervision, guidance and input, to start addressing the finding of the diagnostic phase and to design new ways of working, started to come together. One of the key changes was to simplify the input of referrals, improving the input accuracy from 45 percent to 99 percent overnight. As a result, the validating stopped. The administrators gained huge confidence, not only from now getting it right, but from the fact that they – not Mel, not management – had designed the new process which was now delivering results.

I had to gain sufficient headlines from the weekly meetings to be able to satisfy the constant requests for information from the executive and demonstrate we were moving in the right direction.

I felt we were now ready for the team to go and present to the executive.

Tricia, the admin team lead, and Mark, the booking clerk who had been berated by Gavin so harshly the first time Mel had visited the admin office, rang nervously on the bell to the locked Executive Corridor. "I've never been through these doors before," said Tricia . I didn't want to think how this would have felt if the first time they had come to meet the executive was to be told how badly they were doing and have their "feet held to the fire".

Tricia and Mark stood in front of a packed Committee Room of over 20 senior leaders in the organisation, to share the outcome of their work. I could see Tricia's hand shaking as she started the first slide of her presentation, and heard the wobble in her voice. I think I was as nervous as they were! I caught her eye and gave a big smile. Once they started telling their story, the presentation just flowed. They shared how they had created a paper-free admin office and changed the referral process from random storage of referrals in 48 places to one; how referrals were now received in a single place and scanned within 12 hours; and how they managed their own daily updates of all information and data. They explained this meant they worked with live accurate information, entered correctly first time into their systems, and thus avoided rework or validation. They described the visual management (Mel's Lean background was a key influence here) which informed daily team meetings and work planning they undertook as a team to manage the workload and processes. They shared the improvement trajectory they had developed to plot the performance of the department and demonstrate when they would be compliant with all waiting time targets. So far, they were achieving this in line with the trajectory.

I didn't need to present, nor could I have done. This was their work, developed and owned by them. The leaders and executive team were seriously impressed, "Can you come and do the same for us in cardiology?" one asked.

Learning to see

At the beginning, I struggled to write this story and feel that I deserved to have a place in the exploration of the technical aspects of improvement, because I kept thinking "This isn't my story; this isn't my improvement, I didn't do it". I felt a bit of a fraud that whilst the improvement had happened in my area, I couldn't talk with any confidence about the detail of the work, exactly what had happened, the detail of all the techniques that had been applied. I certainly couldn't replicate it elsewhere. If all I did was to get in an expert in improvement work, how can this be my story about leadership of improvement? And in that struggle, I see some of my leadership story.

When I started I was told "You can do your improvement stuff once you sort the performance out". There was a notion that "doing your improvement stuff" was a separate activity, and equated to being the person who brings the specialist detailed knowledge about improvement methodologies, leading the workshops, being the expert. Maybe this puts some leaders off, as it assumes that deep technical expertise and/or time is required.

Isaacs (1999) talks about leadership as intervention. For me, choosing to lead meant moving from spectating and commenting on situations to active participation and choiceful intervention. Heifetz and Linsky (2002) describe the concept of "getting on the balcony" to allow some reflexive observation of what is happening, and then subsequently returning to the dancefloor to affect what is happening by asking questions, offering praise, listening and drawing attention to what is going on in the moment. These are relational rather than technical skills.

In this situation, my role was not to be the improvement methodology expert, but to create the conditions within which these improvements could occur. It meant providing the team with the additional skills and capacity of Mel to make the necessary improvements; it meant providing the air cover to allow them to do the improvement work away from the constant interruption, judgement, questioning and distraction of the exec teams, who themselves were under significant pressure and were desperate for a solution. What it didn't mean was shouting at people, telling them to get it sorted.

One evening at the end of the day, I wandered up to the admin office to pop my head round the door and say goodbye. When I got there, most of the team had gone home, and Tricia and Mel were sitting in the office, the phones strangely quiet and the room devoid of those teetering piles of paper. "We've been thinking about why this was all so difficult before," said Tricia, "and we have decided that we can write a book on how to make sure you don't improve; it's all the ways we were running the department!" "What do you mean?" I asked, feeling curious, but also a little anxious that they were going to slate the way I was leading the Division.

"Don't let the teams own their own data," said Tricia. "Tick!" said Mel

"Shout at people when the data doesn't give you the answer you want," said Tricia. "Tick!" replied Mel. "So you're too scared to ask for help anyway," finished Tricia.

"Reward people for staying all night and firefighting the situation to get through the next performance meeting." "Tick!"

"Call people to the Trust exec when they have done something wrong, rather than when they have done something well." "Tick!"

"Don't let people order the equipment they need to do their jobs – like a telephone!" "Tick again!" said Mel.

The structure, processes and cultural norms we were creating melded perfectly into what we, half-jokingly, termed "Improvement Prevention Structures".

There's a Lean expression that resonates with me: "Learning to See". It's actually the title of a value stream mapping book, but the expression really sums up what it's like to be involved in improvement. You learn to see what others struggle to, because they are surrounded by it, day in and day out.

Paying attention to the conditions needed to support improvement can lead to an exploration of the cultural norms and ways of doing things that have slowly evolved over time, not always written down or set out as policy, but just "the way we do things". What I noticed as I reflected on the progress we had made was how many formal policy and structural processes *and* cultural practices were also actively working against the team's efforts to design and implement quality improvement. The organisational context was, in effect, clipping our own wings. My role as a leader of improvement was to create a different culture locally, both structurally and behaviourally. Wishing it to be different, and shouting at people to make it so, does nothing to change the conditions or provide the culture and environment for improvement. We sometimes use the metaphor of finding or creating fertile ground, nurturing and tilling that soil to provide the right conditions. Just as shouting at a flower doesn't make it grow, leadership of improvement requires us to pay attention to the environments we are creating, structurally, emotionally and behaviourally, that allow purposeful and meaningful improvements to occur.

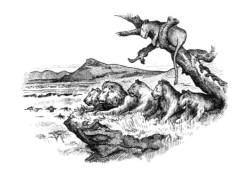

CHAPTER 5

Lessening the Roar

For several years I've been trying! Trying quite hard in fact. Striving to improve patient flow through the children's hospital where I work as a senior clinician. On at least three separate occasions I've led projects designed to enhance flow, specifically by focusing on improving day of discharge percentages. Driven by my own belief and a mountain of evidence that timely patient discharge improves both care quality and flow, I've led these projects with my characteristically robust energy and conviction.

Each time a similar thing happened. Early signs were encouraging, with some significant improvements in key measures. However, after several months things would slowly, inexorably, return to the starting baseline performance. Initial staff enthusiasm turned to frustration and, worse still, cynicism. This led to more general staff resistance about any improvement efforts. Personally I felt a mixture of frustration, failure and annoyance. With each new project I vowed that it would be different, that "This time I'd make it work".

Of course, it never did work. After several years of trying, I came to a rather obvious conclusion. Just doing the same thing and trying harder doesn't work. In fact, it probably makes things worse. The timing of this mini epiphany coincided with me joining the GenerationQ programme, where I had many opportunities for deeper thinking and reflection on my improvement efforts to date. I remember an article by Repenning (2001) on sustaining process improvement that really caught my attention. It helped me understand that simply working harder was not the answer. His idea of not just working smarter but, more importantly, reinvesting in staff to create sustainability was enlightening. I was also struck by his commentary on the "improvement paradox", whereby there are increasing numbers and access to improvement techniques and tools with little evidence of sustained improvement in everyday life. It felt like he understood my world.

Perhaps for the first time I also began to reflect on myself as a leader, and a few doubts set in. I wondered how my "robust energy and enthusiasm" were actually experienced by those around me. Was my well-meaning directness and passion actually getting in the way of progress? Did my colleagues find me overpowering? Looking back on the way our hospital worked, I think that maybe I was partly a product of the culture. The accepted manner for undertaking change was a centralised approach of task and finish. For any given issue the senior team met in private and decided on the best course of action. They then went and spoke to staff about what needed to be done, and expected staff to comply. Failure to deliver was met with more control and direction from management. There was limited dialogue, and staff surveys revealed that people felt "underappreciated", "not listened to", "done to" and "side-lined".

It was sobering to realise that my own style of leading the discharge projects had been quite similar, and I wondered if my own staff felt the same.

This was the impetus for me to try something different. I decided to do a little experimentation.

Ward one: my first experiment

The broad aim of this initiative was very similar to my previous failed QI projects. It was a day of discharge project, looking at midday discharge as a marker.

I'll give a little background. For all the patients clinically ready for discharge on any given day, we looked at the percentage of them discharged before midday. This was seen as a marker of improved efficiency, where an arbitrary level of 30 percent was seen by the Trust as good. There is much evidence to support the view that improving discharge predictability improves flow, quality of care and patient experience (reference NHS Improvement). Within the Trust, many of the wards had traditionally employed extra staff to improve their day of discharge levels. This involved nominated individuals managing processes and trying (often unsuccessfully) to get people to "work harder" and "do the right thing".

I gathered a small team around me, including my Operations Director and a senior and well-respected nurse. Reflecting on my past failures to achieve sustainable change, we were concerned about how the project would be perceived. Would it be seen as "just another project" or "another management idea doomed to failure"? We decided to start small, start slowly, and be almost stealth-like in our approach. We began with just one surgical ward. We decided that for the first two months our only aims were to have conversations with each staff member on the ward, and to begin collecting some data. We resolved that we were not going to make any changes within this time frame. This felt rather counter-cultural and a world away from the typical NHS pressure for action and improvement now!

Importantly, we banned the word *project.* I reflected that my previous attempts had always been termed as projects. Not only did they now have a bad name, it carried several negative connotations – including being done to, pre-determined solutions rolled out, and unrealistic targets in an improbable timeframe. We chose to begin every initial conversation with staff by telling them that this was not a project but an experiment. Our aim was simply to collect data, to try and understand together what could be done to improve the day of discharge rate. There were no targets, processes or pre-determined outcomes.

Our experience showed that not having a target or more clearly defined aim at the outset was immensely beneficial. It allowed us to have many more open conversations with the whole range of staff on the ward, and led to some pivotal moments. For example, this conversation between me and a group of ward staff:

Me: "What do you find most difficult or dislike about working on this ward?"

Nurse 1: "Large numbers of patients arriving every morning for surgery, when the truth is we don't know whether there will be a bed available. It's so stressful for us, and families are often angry – I don't blame them, I would be too..."

Me: "What would be a possible solution?"

Nurse 2: "If only we could predict how many beds we would have each day then we could give far more accurate information to families. We could admit and treat more children. Everything would be simpler and less stressful."

Me: "What would happen if you could more accurately predict whether a child was going to be discharged on any given day?"

There was a long silence in the room, before the nurse replied.

Nurse 2: "....so this is not about day of discharge. It's about accurately predicting who we can admit."

It seems so simple now, but from that point on everyone present completely understood and bought in to what we were collectively trying to achieve. The prize was obvious – less stress, happier families, improved care.

Staff members took the lead, and over the next few months designed and tested a number of simple steps to improve discharge planning and, as a consequence, bed capacity prediction. The role for the team and me was increasingly at arm's length – we were there to support, coach and encourage. Without going into too much detail I'll give you a flavour of what the team did. It's worth saying here that the broad rationale for much of what we ended up doing was informed by the Theory of Constraints (TOC) [See Chapter 2 for more about TOC].

Perhaps the most important data we collected was around reasons for delayed discharge. We measured both whether a child was discharged on time and if they weren't, the reason why not. If a child went over their date of discharge for medical reasons (if they were still sick) then this could not be seen as a failure to discharge on time. We were clear that people would not be held accountable for breaching – we were simply trying to *understand* what was going on.

Interestingly, the reasons staff gave for delayed discharge often bore no relationship to the actual data that was collected. The data gathering process definitely challenged some long-held assumptions. Maintaining curiosity and not seeking to apportion any blame was crucial in these early stages. After the first few weeks we could see some clear patterns around failure to discharge, and staff started creating processes to manage the main constraints.

There were fantastic examples of staff creating innovative solutions. One morning, I came onto the ward to discover each set of patient notes had a card on the front with the processes required to move from admission to discharge for each child. When I asked about this, the staff member remarked: "We have talked amongst ourselves, and we have decided that the only way we can be sure that each child is discharged on time is to be able to see the processes that are needed." I remember feeling delighted. Not only did this perfectly fit with my emerging understanding of TOC, but also the initiative had come from the ward staff with no direction from me.

I recall a conversation I had with a nurse who said: "Being able to see the causes of why children aren't going home on time has allowed me to concentrate on those I have control over. This has definitely stopped me from doing unnecessary work and made my day easier." This ability to see the wood from the trees and actively decrease their workload has certainly encouraged staff to further engage.

After a few months we saw sustained improvement, and amongst the ward staff there was real excitement. The focus changed to how they could not only predict the day of discharge, but the time of day. In addition, there were many other ideas for improving flow and care on the ward that were not related to the initial work.

Together we achieved excellent results. Day of discharge rates more than doubled from 16 percent to 35 percent. We were able to prove a 20 percent increase in patients admitted per month for the same expenditure. Crucially, this improvement was maintained over an extended period of time. This was in stark contrast to my earlier attempts.

We noted a significant uplift in staff mood and morale. The primary reason they gave was that they had the permission to make changes when they encountered problems, without having to go through some lengthy approval process. They felt engaged and trusted, and this was fostering a different local culture.

As one nurse said, "The ability to make changes means that I no longer feel out of control. We have been able to treat more children and we no longer have loads of children waiting to come in. That makes me happy." Unsurprisingly, patients reacted well, with the vast majority of parents and children interviewed talking positively of their experience.

The project had become one that the whole organisation could buy into. From a Trust management perspective it was meeting the targets of day of discharge. It was improving flow of patients, which meant more patients were being treated, and from a staff perspective it was decreasing stress and improving patient experience.

Ward two: repeating the experiment – what could possibly go wrong?

Buoyed by our progress, six months after the initial experiment we started to look at another ward. This time we chose a non-surgical ward where there were familiar discharge issues. As a team we felt that we had learned lots from our work with the surgical ward, so our confidence was high. As we were to discover, confidence can be a dangerous thing! Not wanting to change a successful recipe, we employed exactly the same approach as we had on the first ward. We talked about experimentation not a project, we didn't have (overt) targets, and we took time to engage every staff member in conversation.

Despite using exactly the same methodology and the same support team, we made absolutely no progress. I mean, literally, no progress. After three months there was no improvement in the discharge data. If anything, our presence was making things worse. Ward staff did not seem to be engaged, and some seemed to be actively resisting our efforts.

As a team, we had the presence of mind to pause and reflect. Thank goodness we did. If I'm honest I think that in earlier incarnations of myself I may have just blamed the staff, or just pushed harder and harder trying to make something happen. This time we slowed down and asked ourselves "What's going on here?" and "How come it's not working this time?" Crucially, we tried to make the assumption that however resistant (by which I mean sometimes *really* difficult) staff were being, they were acting from a place of good intent, and were expressing some very real concerns. It's quite easy to write this now, but it was really hard at the time.

A couple of things seemed to be going on. Firstly, even though we had no overt targets, we did have a view as to what level of improvement was possible, from our experience on the surgical ward. We also had opinions on what kind of process improvements and actions could be implemented, again from our knowledge of what had worked previously. I'm not sure we even realised at the time, but despite our protestations that this was just an experiment and that we didn't have set targets or pre-planned implementation ideas, it was hard to forget what we already knew. Whilst we were having conversations with the staff, we were already making assumptions about what should be happening. We thought we already had a winning formula. Almost imperceptibly, we had made the shift from inquiring with the staff to advocating solutions to them. We hadn't created a culture where they felt engaged.

Secondly, we made the mistake of not appreciating the different environment and experience of the non-surgical ward. The staff had a very different attitude towards improving flow. Unlike the first ward, they did not have a crowd of families arriving every day, and did not see the same benefits. Improving flow would simply increase their workload. I vividly remember the frustration of one staff member: "All you have done is increase the number of sick children I have to look after each day which makes my life more difficult." We had failed to understand the (completely valid) experience of the staff on this ward, and in so doing had no buy-in for the overall aim of the experiment. We needed to be completely open and transparent if we were going to tap into the good will of the staff.

The whole experience was both sobering and enlightening. I learnt that context matters; that really listening to staff means suspending what I think I know, or what I think ought to happen; that cutting and pasting a successful approach from elsewhere is no guarantee of success. I also began to reflect more on my own power. I'm a senior clinician. I have positional power and I'm known as a "big voice" in the Trust. Was I seen as too powerful to allow staff to really develop their own ideas? If I was serious about empowering others, how could I do this without stepping back completely, which to me would be an abdication of my leadership role?

I took these questions with me into the next round of experimentation.

Our next experiment – sharing positive stories

I was increasingly struck by the stories we were hearing. The positive accounts of success, creativity and energy in the case of the surgical ward. The stories of stress, failure and frustration in the case of the other ward, which left me feeling so dispirited. I rediscovered what we all know as humans, that stories are incredibly powerful. At this time I also became really interested in something called Appreciative Inquiry (AI) [See Chapter 2 for more about this approach]. Although I found parts of the theory a little philosophical (I am still an impatient medic at heart after all), it helped make sense of what I'd experienced in the first two experiments. Namely, that focusing on what works, and exploring how to do *more* of what works, appears to yield tangible results *and* improve mood and wellbeing. I was acutely aware of how different this was to the dominant deficit-based thinking we encounter in so many parts of the NHS on a daily basis.

We wondered how we could encourage more positive conversations in the Trust generally, away from the specific discharge work we'd been doing so far. Again we wanted to avoid any mention of the *project* word. I firmly believe that attempting to launch some kind of mandatory appreciative storytelling initiative would have been the kiss of death.

I had heard of an American institution where people gathered once a week and talked about what had gone well in the last week, and what they would like to do in the following week to improve patient or staff experience. They then discussed their ideas amongst themselves, chose a couple, and went and experimented. This seemed like exactly what we were after. The idea of using positive conversations to engage staff and give them a safe space to talk and experiment, but more crucially the idea of empowering staff to take ownership without the need to ask for permission.

We started these conversations with the consultant body in a very low-key way, with the invitation to "come along if you're interested". Starting from a positive viewpoint did not mean relentless optimism; more that we are all doing the best we could and should celebrate that. However, in addition we asked ourselves what would we like to do together to make things even better? This drew my attention to the fact that nearly all of our regular meetings are deficit based, starting with the view that everything is a problem to be solved.

For me the most significant learning was just how much was being done under the radar that was brilliant, but no one knew about, because we hadn't stopped and asked. I also noticed that as we started to engage more positively, my fellow consultants seemed to engage more positively in return.

We were hugely encouraged, and decided to try a similar approach on a couple of wards with primarily nursing staff and allied health professionals. In retrospect, this would have been better with all ward staff, but we took a pragmatic approach given that it would be too difficult to get everyone together. We aimed to start small and build.

Without going into a long story, there was a sense of déjà vu from our first two experiments, in that there was both success and failure. On one ward we noticed the remarkable energy, excitement and practical improvements that can emerge from sharing positive stories and working together to design changes. There seemed to be real cultural shift, and staff started to talk about "new possibilities", "a shift in attitude", and "a happier environment". On another ward any initial interest seemed to fizzle out, and the process of weekly ward meetings soon died an untimely death.

In trying to make sense of this, I reflected that sustained change does require real energy and passion from a few people *within* the ward. I'd learnt by this point that I couldn't *drive* change from my senior position. Rather my role seemed to be more about participating, engaging and supporting, and that this helped create a safe place for others to get involved and experiment.

The necessary drive and perseverance has to come from staff. Looking back I can clearly see that the successful ward had a couple of key staff (not necessarily the most senior) who took on a leading role in encouraging their colleagues and, most importantly, keeping going. It reminded me that change takes time, and it's easy to become discouraged and give up too quickly.

Making sense….. with the benefit of some distance

As I re-tell these stories, I find myself reflecting on the most important lessons for me. I'll present these around two main themes: the use of data and QI models, and some reflections on my leadership. These are certainly not definitive conclusions, but rather my current work in progress.

Data and QI models

Data really matters. I've have had many discussions with clinicians about data over the years. Most of them begin: "The data is wrong, therefore...". I was acutely aware how my Trust and most staff viewed data collection and usage. Data was used primarily for accountability or research rather than for improvement. I think it's fair to say there is often fear associated with data collection.

Yet data is the essential starting point in an improvement process. We have to know what is really going on, and this has to be shared amongst everyone, without fear of blame. It involves having the courage to challenge long-held assumptions. For example, at the start of our first experiment we asked staff what was the most common reason patients were delayed in discharge. There was unanimous agreement that radiology and pharmacy caused all the delay. Following data collection, we met again to discuss our findings. The primary reason for delay was that no one had told the family the child was going home the following day! It seems absolutely extraordinary, but it was true.

The use of continuous data collection and sharing is essential to support teams in owning any change. The use of Shewhart charts [see Chapter 2] permits differentiation between causes that signify normal variation and those that have special causes. This allows staff to take control by self-monitoring and dealing with issues that are pertinent and not just background noise.

Of course there will be much conversation around data validity – how it is collected, who collects it, over what timescales, and so on. My reflection now is that defending the rigour of data is often rather pointless. It's far better to ask staff to analyse and make sense of it themselves. I've learnt that the real power of data lies in its ability to start a conversation – a conversation about what is actually happening, and what might be possible in the future. Data is a starting point, not an end point.

In terms of QI methods, I've learnt that a model such as TOC provides a useful structure for understanding where to focus improvement efforts. It also allows us to create some boundaries to work within safely. This is essential if we are going to enable people to experiment with ideas wisely. It's a balance between having enough rules and structure to allow people to feel safe, whilst at the same time encouraging freedom and innovation.

I've also learnt that a method in itself is not sufficient for success. The success of an initiative is not dependent on the improvement theory. I believe that success is dependent on the conversations that occur. With that in mind, storytelling is an essential part of improvement. It is the stories we tell that give meaning as much as the quantitative data we collect. One of my regrets is not having included families in the work. They would have given a richness and different perspective that would have been invaluable, potentially allowing a true co-creation of improvement ideas.

My leadership

I do hope that I am now much more aware of my own impact on others, though I suspect I still have moments of blindness. I think I'm still "robust and passionate" but maybe a little more able to moderate my behaviour and not take centre stage.

Letting go of some power and control

A major reflection is the need to personally let go. The only way to be part of something sustainable is to create the environment where staff genuinely feel empowered. To do this I need to relinquish control, allow people to make mistakes and maybe come to a different answer to the one I initially wanted. I've found this both terrifying and exhilarating simultaneously. Paradoxically I'm discovering that the most powerful thing I can do as a leader is to make myself a little less powerful, to lessen the roar.

This requires bravery on my part, and at times my own anxieties about performance and control made this difficult. I guess that if I am expecting bravery from those around me to make changes, then I have to model that myself. I've discovered bravery is made easier through *authenticity*. An ability to be true to myself, an acceptance of my own weaknesses and a willingness to show vulnerability have been difficult but immensely powerful. I have been able to discuss my fears of failure and need for control at meetings. I've felt less anxious, I feel less of a "Parent", and my colleagues seem to respect me more for it.

Slowing down to speed up

I'm becoming more aware of my own patterns of behaviour that get in the way. In particular, I have a big Hurry Up driver. I hate delay and procrastination in all areas of my life. I have often tried to rush people. In the Trust I would attempt to force or push conversations. Even worse, sometimes I'd just disappear to do other things, citing time pressures. This meant I was not always fully present in the conversation. If, as I believe, change occurs through a myriad of social interactions, then me being fully emotionally and intellectually present in conversations is essential. I need to take more time listening to others; I need to accept that the result may not be perfect, or indeed what I want. I have noted that when I concentrate on these aspects, the tone and quality of the conversation changes. There is increased stillness and more reflection between people, including myself.

This is problematic within the NHS, where projects are often undertaken rapidly and immediate evidence of success is demanded. I am aware that I have been caught within this trap. I have learnt the need to slow down, participate and wait before taking purposeful action. I've also learnt that action can just be an experiment, it doesn't have to be the fully structured plan.

What empowering really means

During our initial experiments, we consciously did not appoint someone to formally lead the change. The closest we had to a project manager was a nurse, well known to the staff on the wards. Her primary role was to talk to families and staff about what they saw and felt, and explain a little about what TOC could offer. We noticed over the first few months that junior nursing staff started to make changes within the ward to speed up discharge. As they noted issues through the data collection, they self-corrected. I remember vividly the first time we saw that staff had developed the additional process discussed above, which noted all the steps needed to get patients to discharge. When we asked why they were doing it, the nurse replied: "This allows us to spot if something has not been done on time." When we asked who had given them permission, there was genuine surprise: "But this is the right thing to do – who do we need to get permission from?" I remember feeling delighted, and saying so.

This appears so counter-cultural within a hierarchal NHS system where waiting for permission is commonplace. I realised it was down to me, as a senior leader, to set a different tone to create a culture conducive to sustained quality improvement. I needed to spend time engaging staff (especially junior staff) to not just agree with what is going on, but truly feel a part of the change; giving them a sense of safety to start experimenting for themselves, without always asking for permission. In a way I cannot directly empower anyone. What I can do, however, is act every day to create a culture where people genuinely feel responsible and can take action without fear. As I write this, it maybe sounds a bit simple and trite – in practice it takes huge patience and presence of mind on my part. I still often get it wrong. Leadership is hard work!

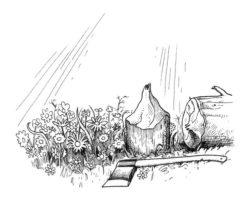

CHAPTER 6

Getting Out of the Way

How much time do you spend in meetings in your working week? I've found it a useful question to reflect on. At one of the workshops on the GenerationQ programme, I was amazed to find that for some leaders it was 90 percent of their time; for clinical leads, like me, it was much less. However, for us too meetings take up a large proportion of non-clinical time. Then there's the next question: What percentage of your time spent in meetings is productive, and how many are you glad you attended? The answer to my own question for me used to be a very low number. Meetings were a good place to catch up on emails, because they were so unengaging.

I am passionate about quality improvement, and in this story I share my own experience of changing the way I lead and participate in meetings, how I approach them now as conversations. It's a story about what I've learned is needed from me to improve the conditions for QI to flourish, and how I've learned about myself personally and have adapted my own leadership style.

The Quality Committee

I had a new job as a medical consultant in a new hospital. I'm generally a high energy, enthusiastic sort of person and was keen to get involved. "No problem," I said, "I will set up and chair the quality improvement committee". I had led some quality improvement work in my old role; I had done several improvement skills training courses, and in my last hospital we had made some good gains. I thought "I can do that again," and "How great to be in a role where I can make things happen".

There was no real steer as to what was expected or what was wanted. I appreciate now that this could have been a real opportunity to develop an innovative and vibrant group. Notice the tense there – could have been...

The first difficulty I encountered was that I was new so I didn't know many people. I certainly didn't know who had any interest, skills or knowledge about quality improvement and safety. I therefore asked the Medical Director, Chief Nurse and Divisional Governance Leads for suggestions. From this I formed a group of doctors and nurses who agreed to meet monthly. Perhaps you have already guessed some of the issues – the usual suspects had been invited; they and I had no personal connection; I only met them when they turned up to the meetings.

I chaired several meetings but, in this new Trust, chairing the Improvement Committee didn't seem as easy as I had first thought. I did as I had done before, but the normal procedures and processes didn't seem to be working. Why not? The improvement work I had led before just didn't seem to be suited for this new role, and the top-down way of delivering the improvement work via committee was not working. As the months went by, nothing seemed to change and actions never seemed to happen. I didn't know what to do to change things. In the end, the meetings just seemed to fizzle out.

I felt very disappointed and, as is my default, assumed it must be down to me as I was the chair. Self-doubt began to creep in. Why was it so easy before, and so difficult this time? Was it me? Why was I not in control of this? Did I not know as much about quality improvement as I had thought? Why did the improvement tools learnt from the Institute for Healthcare Improvement (IHI) and the plan-do-study-act (PDSA) cycles work last time, yet not this time?

Looking back I can see that I chaired the group in quite an authoritative style. I felt I was probably the person with the most expertise in quality improvement and, to be honest, I hadn't thought about my leadership style. I didn't ask about any support that would be needed to develop the ideas that were generated at the Committee Meeting, as I just assumed that the group members would go and lead and make things happen in their individual areas.

I had moved from a small district general hospital, where I knew nearly all of the consultant body and most of the senior nurses, and my approach had worked well there. Here there was much less contact between different specialties in the Trust; silo working was more apparent, and I hadn't appreciated how much harder it was to disseminate information. In my enthusiasm to just get on with the task, I had mentally assumed that plug and play, doing what had worked before, would work again. I hadn't taken into account some of the cultural differences within this much larger Trust, and the need to adapt my approach to this new context. I realised I had been behaving just like a donkey, politically unaware, just doing my own thing without connecting meaningfully with others or adapting to the new environment. I wasn't tuned into the organisational grapevine, and had not been able to develop sufficient relationships. I had no real attachment or affinity for any of the people attending the meeting, or them for me. I knew how to improve my own work but not how to enthuse and support others to improve their work.

Huddles with the quality nurses

As part of GenerationQ, we visited different organisations to see how others implemented different QI techniques and approaches. One visit was to Unipart, the logistics company based in Oxford, whose whole business is based round Lean.

I am attracted to Lean as I find its emphasis on eliminating "muda" ("waste" in Japanese) inherently attractive. Waste in this context means any human activity which absorbs resources but creates no value: mistakes that require rectification; production of items no one wants so that inventories and goods pile up; and time waiting – a team ready to perform surgery but the patient hasn't arrived or patients are waiting. I believe that Lean used at a local level can contribute to improvements within that area, however Lean seems to me to be most effective when it is part of the whole system's drive to continuous improvement, as it was at Unipart. For this to happen, engagement from everyone is required, from the board to the frontline staff. My Trust is not there yet, but I believe the board are open to new ways of working and are keen to foster a culture of improvement, so it feels good to be able to support growing engagement and understanding about QI.

During the Unipart visit, we heard about the informal groups they have that meet standing up, and are called "Our Contribution Counts" (OCC) circles. These seemed quite like the safety huddles that I had used before in my previous role, but in Unipart the huddle was being used in a more generic way, to develop improvement ideas rather than just for safety or handovers. These seemed to have a real energy about them and were very democratic. Members of the huddle in Unipart are involved in the imple-mentation of the quality improvement ideas, and everyone's opinion is important. This is different to the more hierarchical way that health care tends to be delivered, with consultants and matrons making decisions and running their units with little or no input from others on the wards. How might this style of huddle work in a hospital setting? What translation process would be required? (After my bruising experience with the Quality Committee, plug and play without adaptation wasn't something I was going to countenance again!)

Back in the hospital shortly after my visit to Unipart, I heard about some new specialist nursing posts that were being established by the Nursing Director to support quality improvement. I wondered if I would be able to do some work with these quality nurses, given my QI skills and enthusiasm to improve quality. But I was nervous and a bit bruised after the Quality Committee experience. The Nursing Director had a reputation for being intimidating and formidable. What if she thought I was completely bonkers, wasting her time?

I chatted about how to approach her with some GenerationQ colleagues. Thinking ahead about a forthcoming meeting hasn't been my normal approach. Neither has sharing my anxieties with others. However, I've learned that both can lead to me being more choiceful and the outcomes much better.

"What have you got to lose?" said Kate.

"See it as an opportunity to have a conversation," advised Doug.

"Ask her some questions first to find out why she has set up the quality nurses," advised Kumar. "And what about all that stuff we've been reading about dialogue? See it as an opportunity to build the relationship and explore the idea rather than presenting her with a fixed proposal."

I worked up the courage and approached the Nursing Director who, to my surprise, was immediately supportive and not at all scary. Just shows how you can convince yourself something is going to be far worse than it actually is. She was extremely happy for me to work with her team to deliver improvements and to put my technical background in quality improvement to good use. She thought it was also really positive to have a doctor supporting this work, as it symbolically signalled that this was work that everybody should take seriously. She also said that the quality nurses knew much more about quality assurance than quality improvement, so I could share my QI knowledge of the latter with them.

Thinking about my meeting with the Nursing Director, and how enthused and willing she had been to work with me, despite my initial misgivings and her prior reputation, made me wonder what the specialist nurses might think of me when I met them. What might they imagine me to be like? Some consultants have a reputation – busy, arrogant, angry, frustrated, impatient, intolerant and ignorant of the work others do every day. I wondered what I could do to ensure a good first meeting to help us start our work together well, and decided to try and be as open and welcoming as the Nursing Director had been with me.

In one of the books I was reading, Patricia Shaw makes an interesting suggestion: "...maybe the solution is a meeting designed as a prolonged coffee break" (Shaw 2002, p15). I also had Kumar's voice in my head: "Ask, not tell. Think conversation".

I met four of the quality nurses in the Costa near the hospital entrance and bought them all a coffee. This in itself was something that surprised them. When I first mentioned the idea of huddles to the quality nurses, there was a fair amount of scepticism in the room.

"Will ideas from 'the shop floor' actually get listened to?"

"Is this just another gimmick from on high?"

But as we kept talking they seemed to warm to the idea. I made a deliberate effort to get them talking, to find out what they had been doing in their roles as quality nurses and to explore their understanding of the differences between quality assurance and quality improvement. I was trying to meet them where they were at. I then had the first huddle with a group of staff on a geriatric ward with one of the quality nurses attending. There seemed to be a willingness for the staff present to take a lead with their own ideas on how to improve their own working environment. Many of the ideas didn't really tally with the IHI methodology, but appeared to follow a more Lean approach in cutting out waste. I discussed this with a couple of the sisters, who appeared a bit hesitant when I mentioned Lean. I asked a few more questions and they said that they had tried Lean previously with the productive ward initiative. It had worked for a bit, they said, but gradually everything had returned to the status quo. It sounded as though they didn't use all of the five principles, but stopped after the first three. Things had been moved around on the ward after process mapping, waste was eliminated to improve flow but without establishing pull or continuous improvement, so the Lean process was a static, one-off event. Perhaps therefore not a surprise that it didn't become established, not that I said that to them.

It was useful to know about their experience and a salutary reminder that, if you don't ask, you don't know where people are coming from. You don't really meet them where they're at. You don't know their back story and history, so can easily make the wrong assumptions or take negativity personally when it is actually based on a previous experience.

At the end of the meeting they decided that overall, they really liked the concept of huddles, especially that the improvement ideas could come from anyone in the team, rather than just the manager and then filtered down through the hierarchy. This aspect was seen as a bit revolutionary and subversive and they particularly relished it. They were up for it! I was cautious but delighted. If the huddles became established then this could mean that there was a platform for continuous improvement that wasn't previously possible.

The idea we created together was as follows: we would have a short stand up multidisciplinary team meeting as a huddle to come up with ideas to make life easier, using open appreciative questions. The huddle would include the whole clinical team: porters, health care assistants, junior doctors, consultants and matrons. I hoped that, because few of the team members would have been asked before what they could do to help improve things, never mind been given permission, autonomy and support, there would be some traction. This time, I was trying to make sure the improvement ideas would be led by the team, come from the bottom up rather than from me, and I hoped this would lead to more success.

Working this way was a challenge for me personally because, historically, I had always run projects in a very planned and prescribed way. Learning about complexity thinking as part of GenerationQ encouraged me to allow for some experimenting and emergent change.

An example of this was at the first Medicines Management Improvement huddle which took place on a date when I was away, so I couldn't facilitate it. I think previously I would have postponed the first huddle until I could be present. However, I had confidence in the quality nurse who facilitated the huddle, and the group carried out a couple of PDSA cycles and made some significant improvements in the medication error rate on their ward. The quality nurse who facilitated this huddle then went on to facilitate huddles on other wards. This was energising for her. I was delighted, although I admit I had a few twinges of envy, wishing I'd been there. However, I know that this is part of my learning: I don't have to be there as a hero, doing everything or aware of all the fine detail. The results are sometimes not what I expected, but are often greater than I expected. This has also helped with my resilience as a leader, as I can now trust teams and allow them more space.

Looking at what has been emerging from the huddles, many of the ideas can be taken forward using Lean principles; some of the possible ideas generated mirror Lean very closely, and some of the improvement work already happening uses Lean, but is not badged as such. It is less formal than the work I did in my previous Trust, but this seems to work better where I am now, so pragmatism rules OK in my book.

There have been good questions from staff as the huddles have developed. A frequent question is whether there should be patient representatives within the huddle. A valid question, as the patient can be seen as the customer, and Lean principles are driven by what the customer values. Rather than try and legislate on this, we've said that to do so or not depends on the appetite in the different wards. For me personally, the main thing is that the huddles give staff a voice. I heard Richard Branson talking recently and he said, "If you look after your staff, then they'll look after your customers. It's that simple."

And of course not everything that has been tried on the wards has delivered an improvement. One of the aspects I like in the Model for Improvement is the principle that "All improvements require change, but not all change will result in Improvement" (Langley et al 2009, p. 2). Before, I led QI projects from a distance, not involving myself too closely with those on the ward, and I never really thought about the emotional impact of things not working and the possibility of people becoming disheartened. I now try and make sure we talk about this. If a desired improvement doesn't happen, it doesn't mean that it wasn't a success. In the words of Steve Chapman, an expert on creativity, in order to learn, it is important to "Fail Happy". The word failure has many negative connotations. In my context I now often reframe an improvement project that didn't have the desired outcome as a positive attempt where there was much to learn.

Securing funding for an Improvement Academy

To support the work going on in the huddles, I felt we needed to spread quality improvement skills across teams to support their learning and the potential success of the huddle work. I guess the question was really, what was needed to develop the conditions in which the improvement activity could thrive and grow? I knew other organisations were developing Improvement Academies to deliver training across a range of QI techniques and methods, and to create a space and community for teams to meet and learn together to support their endeavours. But to do this, we needed some funding.

Building on my previous learning, I thought carefully about how to approach the Trust board. After my failed attempt to lead the improvement committee, I decided that I couldn't just bring a paper to the board asking for financial support. Instead, I took a relational approach, electing to have one-on-one conversations beforehand to support the formal board paper.

This is something else I have been learning. Don't just meet senior folk in the formal setting of the official meeting – the "front stage". Go and meet them before, back stage, so you know them, you have a sense of what is important to them, and you can have dialogue rather than the set piece presentation to the exec team. This was a strategy that I hadn't used before. Was it the sort of thing real leaders did?

My GenerationQ buddies were useful again:

"Navigating senior relationships and understanding the power and politics is how you shape the ongoing conversations," said Kate.

I emailed the Chief Executive Officer and talked with the Chief Nurse in advance of the meeting, so that they knew about my request beforehand. Their questions also helped to improve the paper. I had originally wanted to set up an academy which included a simulation centre, as well as support for quality and continuous improvement across the Trust, but they were clear the former was too ambitious, so I scaled back to something that felt more do-able. To my delight and surprise we got the go ahead, not quite as much funding as I wanted but still a green light to create a virtual academy. In the meeting the most intense grilling came from the Finance Director. Next time I'll make sure I meet her beforehand too.

Unbeknownst to me, the Finance Director had sponsored a GenerationQ Fellow when she was in her previous Trust, so she was well disposed, despite the grilling. Brian, the Deputy Chief Nurse, has been the other key ally. I have been helped here by knowing him from my previous Trust. The two of them met when I was on annual leave following the board meeting. When I returned, I was informed that the Academy had been approved for funding for a Band 8a (Matron level) project manager to get it up and running, and substantial funding from the Trust's charity to pay for the initial training of the first cohort of the QI trainers in the Academy. It was another lesson in my realising I didn't have to be present for things to move forward.

In the Academy we offer a range of concepts and methodologies, including Theory of Constraints, the IHI Model for Improvement, Lean and Six Sigma. One of the key purposes of the Academy is to develop a faculty trained in these technical skills, especially in the IHI methodology, and with the theory of Lean. Now that I have learned about complexity thinking, I have a different way of understanding how change actually happens. Even in the early stages, setting up the Academy didn't follow a straightforward linear path, and what is developing is very different to what I initially envisaged, and will undoubtedly change again as it develops. Two years ago I would probably have felt frustrated at this or even seen it as a personal failure. Now I see change as a more emergent process, recognising that some things are outside of my or the Trust's control. Recently, I feel I have made an important move: rather than myself or Brian chairing the Steering Group for the Quality Academy, we've given the role to Emma, the project manager. Other than the data analyst, Emma has the least positional power, but by allowing her to chair the group she has ownership of the work, which feels right, as she is the only full-time member of staff working on the Academy, and so potentially has the most invested in it. Giving her the chair I hope will give her more confidence to experiment and develop the Academy.

Revisiting the huddles

The initial improvement huddle experiments seemed to work quite well, especially when we supported them with experienced facilitation together with an appreciative approach. However, the improvement huddles didn't seem to "take off" quite as I had imagined, even with the Academy support and training. About a year in, I had a long conversation with the nursing team about how effective the improvement huddles were. We had some good ideas and projects, but when the expert facilitator left the circles to self-facilitate, they seemed to struggle, and finding time to take part suddenly became difficult. It seemed like the radical and bottom-up approach of asking staff to come up with improvement ideas was too difficult to enact within the innate hierarchical context of the NHS. Staff were so used to being told what to do, they were still waiting to be told what to do! And I suppose it was scary; it was scary for me to act differently, so I think it was also very scary for everyone else too.

The nurses involved suggested that the lack of focus for the huddles, without a specific improvement aim, was in their view part of the reason for the difficulties. This was a difficult conversation for me, as I had put so much energy into their development, and the original idea had been to ensure the improvement huddles were more open rather than standardised and topic focused. I could feel myself being annoyed, but I decided this would be unhelpful and I needed to be flexible. Rather than stick to the original improvement huddle format, I agreed with the team to try out more focused huddles, even though this seemed a little like a top-down approach. These have been much more successful; the number of improvement ideas have measurably grown from different staff groups, there appears to be much more ownership for the completion of actions, and we have stronger relationships. It seemed to change our conversation. "Aha," I thought, "Perhaps it is about the unique blend of top-down and bottom-up change that is needed, rather than one or the other."

There are still challenges; whilst I feel we have secured support from the board and the managerial community – which has enabled us to train over two hundred improvement learners – medical, rather than nursing support is not really there. To tackle this, I established a similar improvement training process for junior doctors and foundation trainees to support and encourage quality improvement from the bottom up. Interestingly, I've been helped by a change in the external context: my medical college now requires all our senior medical trainees to take part in quality improvement projects as part of the process to become consultants. Registrars must now learn the technical elements of improvement, and about working with stakeholders, and reflect on their successes and failures during their projects. This has led to some ambitious improvement projects, such as the redesign of some care pathways to improve care. It is also interesting because we are facing the same problem with this activity as we did with the nurses: it is difficult to choose what to work on and to sustain the activity when key individuals leave, and it becomes exhausting when there are so many other pressures on your time.

Building on the learning from the improvement huddles, I am blending top-down support with bottom-up ideas, being careful to not overpower and cause imbalance between the two. I am introducing some structure to help choose the improvement projects and to ensure formal handover of work between doctors when their placements rotate. In many ways, this helps us, as an organisation, to own these improvement projects as much as the individual doctors in training do. This increase in prioritisation and focus is also helping to manage our time pressures and to collaborate and share learning across departments better. I feel we are also becoming more open in our reporting and risk management activity.

I am now recognising that whilst we can develop the environment where teams of staff can take part in improvement activity, and have the skills and support to do it, individuals still need to want to do it. Individuals must choose to take the opportunities themselves; I can't make them do that. I have had to learn to accept that, because if I tell them to do it – that is, "You have to come up with improvement ideas in this improvement huddle, rather than me," then how is that any different? Ironically, this would just be another way to lead via diktat. I have learnt that my role is to create a safe space for teams to try out their improvement ideas and to encourage and support that activity, to console when the ideas don't work, and to celebrate loudly when they do. I will know we are successful when you can walk into any department or ward and staff on those wards can demonstrate their improvements, and can talk about the work that is ongoing, ideas they have to improve, and the new improvement concepts they are currently trialling as part of their routine daily activity, not as part of special projects.

I started this chapter by accepting an improvement leadership position that I thought would be straightforward. I thought improvement was all about tools and techniques, about driver diagrams, measurement and flow charts. This stuff is important but in the end, for me, this is not what improvement is about. Improvement is all about my relationships and my conversations. The tools and techniques just help to frame the conversations and systematise them, and a skilled improver knows both when to, and crucially when not to, use them within their conversations. Improvement is talking to people and building a conversation across the organisation about how to make things better, together, top down and bottom up. Without the conversations, nothing happens. That to me has turned out to be much more important than the improvement tools and techniques.

And for me personally, I'm much happier. I have the confidence to have conversations, to knock on an exec's door, regardless of the hierarchy. I worry less if I don't know what to do and I am happier listening to ideas from other people. I also worry less if it doesn't work. I can let things emerge and change, and perhaps more importantly I don't need to be "at the top". I don't feel that I need a role to lead improvement or to have all the answers myself. Instead I can go with my colleagues wherever the improvement work takes us together.

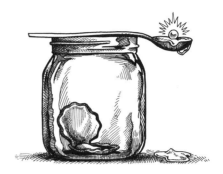

CHAPTER 7

Moving through Treacle, Discovering Pearls

I am first in. I'm in a new role and supposed to be the Medical Director. Pamela, the Managing Director, arrives a few minutes later looking stressed and hurried, flings her trench coat over the back of a chair and takes a seat at the PC next to me. She straightens her back, breathes in and as she does so she pulls her tailored box jacket down lightly but firmly. Unexpectedly Dave, the Nursing Director, arrives almost immediately afterwards and, holding a piece of toast, sits down next to her. "Morning," he says.

We both respond cheerily but without looking up. We are in a line, side by side, tapping on our keyboards and staring ahead at our monitors.

Then, distracted by a thought, I say, "Anyone actually got to grips with this joint accountability thing I keep being told about? Still don't get how it's meant to work."

Pamela stops typing for a moment, looks up, pushes her chair back. "Yeah, well actually that's not what we're being told. We, I mean the other Managing Directors and me, we're being told these divisions are like 'mini-Trusts', and to think of our roles as mini-CEOs," she says.

"No," says Dave, "Joint..... That's definitely been the operative term in my conversations too. Christ, do they actually know their arses from their elbows?" he chuckles. "At least I know for sure that all us nurses, we're leading on quality. Suits me."

"No but the Medical Directors are doing quality."

"No, what I heard is you lot are doing the assurance."

"No, that's us," says Pamela. "Performance and assurance is definitely us."

Pamela's mobile begins to buzz persistently. She dives into her bag and wanders away muttering urgently, her hand cupped to her mouth. Dave catches sight of his watch, kicks back his chair and declares, "Oops, meeting, five minutes ago!" rushing away. Another email drops into my mailbox.

Sitting there trying to compute this conversation, I'm feeling as if I am thinking through a light swirling mist, and notice that I'm a little riled. Then I begin to chuckle as something dawns on me: maybe someone somewhere is trying to implement complexity thinking [see Appendix 1] without telling us? I'm on the GenerationQ Leadership programme, and have begun to find it helpful to think with Stacey's (2012) ideas about organisations not as machines with structures, but something more emergent, made up only of interactions between people, fleeting and myriad individual gestures and the responses to these gestures. That could feel like chaos, I think, and that's actually exactly how it feels to me right now.

Then I resign into a deep sigh. I conclude at least that if the three of us are this confused then our colleagues must be confused too; probably even more so. I resolve to get out and meet people, see how they are faring in their different departments, teams and services. I am craving activities and conversations that feel more creative, purposeful and constructive, and I hope they will be too. As I will share in the story that follows, I had a good idea about what I was aiming for but I had not anticipated all that I was about to learn.

Every good story has a beginning, a middle and an end. So let's begin.

The beginning

I had been appointed as a medical director, though not in the executive team, of "Wilderness Health", a large Trust with multiple sites that had grown exponentially through an ambitious and successful acquisition strategy. The story takes place at the beginning of an enormous redesign programme, the second in four years, as the organisation is also simultaneously reacting to an apparently unanticipated financial crisis. In the previous structure, lines of accountability had seemed reasonably clear, but as multiple new acquisitions were made these had been feeling increasingly unwieldy. The response was to merge and reorganise the numerous old directorates to create four new divisions, each led by a divisional triumvirate: a nursing, medical and managing director.

I had come to my new post with a track record for delivering improvements, and had always worked on projects closely with staff from all sorts of professional backgrounds, and also with many patients and carers. My commitment to quality improvement is fuelled by deeply held personal values about inclusion, diversity, and participation. I am motivated by the idea of organisational life as rich and diverse as the communities for whom health and social care are provided. I was feeling pleased with what I had achieved in previous roles, and at the same time ready for a new challenge. So I too was in a transition of my own.

I had also recently been introduced to a new improvement approach called the Theory of Constraints (TOC) [See Chapter 2]. Applied in a health care setting, this theory proposes that the progress of a patient through any care pathway is a series of dependent events. As one of my GenerationQ colleagues likes to say, the journey along the pathway is only ever as good as the weakest link. I was drawn to the way in which TOC begins from a basic assumption about the inevitability and significance of interdependencies in work. Since the theory is premised on the idea of a system, adjustments in work in one part of any system require adjustments throughout. For me, TOC suggests not only a way of measuring improvement, but also a philosophy of organisational work that I felt complemented my leadership approach. It offers a practical strategy for improvement, but is also a sort of management philosophy. I like the emphasis it places on the importance and value of effective team working

With a strong desire to expand the quality improvement capability of the workforce, and wanting also to instil more of a sense of shared purpose and team-working, I set out to visit each directorate and find out what was going on.

I met with all my clinical directors, including Clive. He had been part of a directorate management team for several years and, in the previous organisational structure, had reported directly into the executive. I knew he and his colleagues were particularly unhappy about the re-structure, and so I wanted him to come alongside to work with me on quality improvement. After some initial pleasantries, the discussion went something like this:

"It's a mess! Total mess." He is shaking his head back and forth vigorously. "A new structure, yet another one; no-one understands what the hell's going on or who's doing what."

"Yes, it's created lots of uncertainty and disruption, I know," I say.

"Even more tiers of bl***dy management costs than before!" he continues.

"Hard to believe I know that it's saved on costs. And I know it's been really disruptive," I mutter consolingly.

"You're an overhead! We didn't need you then and we don't need you now." He leaves abruptly.

Within seconds, I found myself wishing I had said or done something different, but was unsure what. Perhaps you have been there too? I could accept that people were finding the pace and scale of organisational change hard, but I was also thinking, "Is this really how people have been accustomed to talking and behaving?" I had been taken off guard. I was feeling annoyed.

As I continued my visits, I developed a hunch that in one particular directorate, the City Services, relationships between frontline staff and their managers were working reasonably well. Perhaps they would be ready for a more in-depth discussion about quality improvement work? I decided to just get on with it and organise an event where we could play the Dice Game, which I'd enjoyed at a past GenerationQ workshop, as a way of experientially demonstrating the principles of TOC.

My aim was to design an event to stimulate more awareness of quality improvement as a method. I wanted it be open to anyone who was interested to learn, irrespective of their professional background or seniority. I hoped we might even manage to identify some specific projects reflecting the frontline's redesign priorities. I hoped the meeting could feel like a place where people were listening to each other, sharing concerns and finding solutions together. Could I encourage a more open, inclusive and conversational style of meeting? Could operational and clinical staff, old and new, corporate and local, all work together even if for only two or three hours? Could we develop together a sense of a common purpose to improve the quality of our patients' care?

I decided to play the Dice Game, a game designed to illustrate some important principles of TOC. Players are grouped into teams and sit in a row to simulate a production line or pathway. Each team player has one dice and a pile of counters. The counters represent patients moving along the care pathway, and the dice represents statistical variation that arises from all the unpredictable occurrences that arise day to day, at each work station. Theoretically, each player or station has the same capacity for work, varying from one to six depending on the roll of the dice. If each player rolls, let's say, a four then work would flow seamlessly from one work station to another along the production line. Of course, this never happens. Some players in the line throw high, some low, and this changes with each throw of the dice. Flow through the system varies accordingly. The game demonstrates that each work station along any production line is a dependent event, with the result that bottlenecks build up and move along the line and between stations unpredictably. A perfectly formed production line is a beautiful idea, but with life in a complex world only variation is constant. Bottlenecks, or queues, are inevitable and managers will never know where the next bottleneck will emerge. Throughput goes up and down constantly with all the implications for wasted resources, reduced quality and extra costs. What is needed to increase the capacity of the pathway? The game points to an answer: concerted effort to effectively manage the most significant bottleneck in the system at any given time.

I can remember the event as if it was happening now:

> *In preparation for the workshop itself, I pay a lot of attention to stakeholder engagement, to the back stage. Given my commitment to inclusion I am surprised to notice an unmistakable impulse to leave out Pamela and Dave, my co-directors in the triumvirate. With all this confusion going on, wouldn't that just be so much simpler, I think to myself? Simultaneously, I am also wondering if these dilemmas about inclusion or exclusion reflect on wider, systemic issues that are now being played out between myself and my colleagues. Am I justified in mistrusting their ambitions? Or am I just experiencing a sense of personal rivalry toward them? To answer these questions, do I need to learn more about the system and the people I'm working with, or more about myself?*

> *At the very least, I am learning that as a leader I need to stay aware of my own feelings. So I resist the temptation to act on them and decide to park them, to keep them in mind. I remind myself that by initiating the event I'm making a significant move or gesture as a leader with this new group of people, and I want to embody the values that are important to me. So, I personally invite Dave and Pamela and do my best to persuade them the meeting will be worth their while. For now, at least, I feel satisfied that I have ensured the event starts off from a stance of inclusivity.*

> *To encourage all manner of people from across the service to attend, I begin by securing the commitment of more senior colleagues and local managers; I draw on their suggestions about who to invite to make sure we have as diverse a group of junior managers and different specialties and roles as possible. I am trying my best to develop a constituency of the willing and interested in finding ways of improving quality. I have lots of conversations, some short, others longer, being open and explicit about my intentions, about why I am doing things in this way. I hope the initiative will be seen as genuinely involving others in creating shared power structures that complement more existing formal power structures, not as attempts to usurp them. I tread thoughtfully, carefully, purposefully onwards.*

> *Twenty-four hours before the engagement event, I have no idea if these plans will work and virtually no idea who will come. By nine*

o'clock the following morning, I am relieved that there are already 25 people in the room. More drift in over the minutes that follow. I have prepared chairs and tables in a circle around the edges of the room. I have put bowls of fruit and biscuits on the two long tables I have set up for the game. In the GenerationQ programme I've also been learning about what it takes to create the conditions for people to genuinely connect, paying attention to the invitation beforehand, to the setup of the room. It's not that you can, or want, to control what will happen but you can "till the soil". In this way, I provide some nurture and wait to see what might germinate and take root.

There are huge piles of large colourful counters at the head of each table. I have a whistle. I am aiming to create an atmosphere that is noisy, playful and a little competitive. Once everyone has introduced themselves, I outline the workshop plan. I'm aiming to work with the spontaneity and positivity that can be generated by playing games, to loosen people's familiar groupings and encourage them to associate with one another in new ways, to connect, to be relational. By providing a relatively unstructured space for dialogue immediately afterwards, I actively enable a dialogue with everyone gathered in the room.

When everyone is ready, I say, "On my count of three, throw your dice and move the corresponding number of patients' counters through your work station and onto the next. OK? Throw!"

I blow the whistle!

After a momentary pause, the attentive silence in the room is broken up by the soft rattling of rolling dice. The murmuring of voices gets gradually louder as comments, questions and exclamations emerge.

"Hang on. Help! Which way do we move the counters again? Towards you?"

"No, to your right. That way."

"Hello, here, have some work from me. Four for you! Having a particularly productive day." He pushes along a pile of counters to his right.

"Four! Well thank you very much. Got quite a pile here. Ha! Must be what they call a bad hair day for me! I can't seem to move enough of it on. I need some sixes!"

The session is very interactive and it feels like we've all had some fun. Before calling time, I establish there is an appetite for further meetings like this. I bring the event to a close by thanking everyone and

distributing an evaluation sheet. Once the room is empty, I read the
written feedback. I feel the stirrings of excitement and some
trepidation. Did it work for them? Could this be the start of something?
I read, "I am the team manager of Buttercup Ward. Really interesting
and good fun! I want to use this approach to reduce the length of stay
in my unit." Another says, "Fantastic! I thoroughly enjoyed meeting
people and having the chance to talk about what we think about
changes in future!" I can see opportunities opening up for more
quality improvement work. I am thrilled.

The middle

Elsewhere in the division, my interactions were feeling less up-lifting. With my divisional team colleagues, I was finding it challenging to develop a sense that we were working as any sort of team. So, I just carried on doing what I could to strengthen these relationships and clarify team working within my trio of co-directors as well as the divisional management teams. I noticed how the atmosphere could quickly become hostile, uncooperative, even disrespectful and I felt the best I could do was to take steps to broker more open, honest relationships. I keep in mind that TOC as an approach is underpinned by the philosophy that continuous brokering, negotiating, and dialogue is essential if the system is to continue to work well. Without this engagement a greater or lesser degree of derailment becomes inevitable. The dice game makes this manifest, visually, experientially, elegantly.

By now, I had also had one-to-one meetings with all of the clinical directors in the divisional management team. Each of them had used these meetings to voice, to a greater or lesser degree, unhappiness with the re-structure. People asked questions about joint accountability, wanting more clarity about what they could expect from their director trio. I felt uncomfortable that I found these questions so difficult to give a direct answer to. However, I was at least able to begin a discussion about quality improvement. I hoped I could bring each of these directors alongside me in this work.

From the GenerationQ programme, I had begun to make a habit of reflective journalling, making a few notes after some events and interactions that had particularly struck me in some way, helping me to gain a new perspective on my working environment. Regretting the friction and confusion within the divisional trio, I decided to bring this up in a one-to-one discussion with my own manager (Ian), and later I made some notes about what had struck me:

Me: *How's joint accountability meant to work?*

Ian: *You, Pamela and Dave talk about it.*

Me: *I have done, several times. They don't get it either.*

Ian: *Talk to them again.*

Me: *Pamela doesn't want to talk about it. Pamela doesn't really talk about anything.*

Ian: *Talk to Nigel [her boss].*

Me: *Is that a good idea?*

Ian: *Well he's jointly accountable.*

Reflection: *Doing as my manager says = right thing to do. Talking about colleagues to their own manager = wrong thing to do. Result = dilemma.*

A few days later having cautiously followed Ian's advice, I did some more journalling:

Me: *Ian suggested talking to you.*

Nigel: *Sure.*

Me: *It's about joint accountability. Pamela doesn't really talk to anyone.*

Nigel: *Well maybe you need to talk to her about that.*

Me: *I don't think you understood what I just said.*

Nigel: *I'll talk to Ian.*

Reflection: *No-one really understands joint accountability.*

Soon after this meeting, I met Clive again, this time at an appointments panel for a significant position in his directorate. We were joined also by his directorate's operational manager and Pamela, my co-director, who were also panel members. On paper, both candidates appeared reasonably qualified for the post. At the beginning of the interview Clive declared his prior acquaintance with one of the candidates. During the interview, I found this candidate's responses adequate, but his style overfamiliar, leaving me with the impression that he thought the job already his. I was perhaps also feeling more bruised by my recent encounter with some of the clinical directors than at the time I wanted to admit to myself.

When we reached the panel discussion and each member's feedback, the majority view began to emerge in this candidate's favour. However, I found myself feeling strongly that some complacency had set into this discussion, and when my turn came I acknowledged the candidate's strengths and also, unambiguously, my perceptions of his weaknesses and my concerns. This broke the emerging consensus. It felt disruptive, uncomfortable and, frankly, it felt good. I was not surprised when Clive challenged me directly. The chair of the panel picked up on this discord, insisting on further discussion before a decision was reached. I knew very well that I was making an important point and trying to be awkward. Having made Clive and everyone else sweat for a while, I capitulated. The candidate was appointed. I now felt reasonably satisfied with the outcome as well as the process, yet even so I left the meeting feeling stirred up.

Reflecting afterwards, had I been right to assert myself with Clive like this? I thought so, but I also recognised there had been a dollop of my own petulance thrown in. Although I couldn't see clearly at the time, by stealth the drama triangle [see Appendix 2] was beginning to encroach and enfold myself and others. My well-meaning intentions to invest more personally in building some of these relationships were beginning to stall.

The interview panel had also left me more aware of the tensions building between myself and my co-director, Pamela. While we were superficially working together, I was finding her style towards me and others either inaccessible and remote or unduly dictatorial and abrasive. "She is being a mini-CEO," I thought to myself. I wasn't wanting to be in charge myself, to be some lonely heroic leader, but I did want the three of us to agree what we were each in charge of and to work well together, creating the context for others around us to work well together. Soon after this, I decided to tackle these various tensions more directly. I approached Pamela, hoping that by doing so I might engender more of a sense of solidarity, understanding and trust between us.

"I'm feeling so annoyed about yesterday. It takes a lot for me to lose my equilibrium but that's what's happening."

"Personally, I didn't feel that strongly about it," she said, somewhat dismissively.

"I'm just so fed up with Clive. You can probably hear it in my voice right now. It's the attitude, like everything's sewn up, nobody else's business."

"Actually, I know what you mean. I had to speak to him last week and, boy, can he talk down. You know, like he does. Do you know what I said? I said, 'What exactly are you trying to say here, Clive?' And I was thinking, actually, I just haven't got time for this. So eventually I just said, 'Do you know what,

Clive, I'm not asking you. I'm telling you. It's not good enough and I'm telling you to go and sort it out!'"

"Yes, I can just see it."

"If you really want to know what I think, I'll tell you. His directorate manager's a puppy dog and frankly he's a p****."

Although this meeting involved so much more personal disclosure by both Pamela and myself, why then did I leave feeling even more unsettled? On reflection, I think we were colluding in a game of "isn't he awful" in terms of the drama triangle, because in the way he talked down to people Clive had left both of us feeling like victims, despite the fact we were supposed to be more senior! Despite my intentions, we weren't sharing our feelings with the aim of resolving the situation. That is to say we weren't in an "Adult" mode. These relationships around my director role continued to feel messy and uncomfortable.

In contrast, after the Dice Game event, I was feeling much more confident that there were people in the City Services who wanted to learn more about quality improvement. I set up a monthly QI meeting open to anyone to join. In contrast to my experience of a deadening feeling elsewhere, I wanted people to feel valued, respected, creative and involved. I made a point of getting to know Brian, the manager of Buttercup Ward, visiting him and his team on the ward. Buttercup Ward offered older people's mental health care. It had a fixed number of beds for the borough it served, but demand was now outstripping supply. Many patients' discharge was delayed as they waited for suitable support to be arranged for them in the community, and some patients waiting for admission were being placed in similar wards provided by other local authorities.

I asked Brian who he wanted to involve in his project. He suggested Parmjeet the team's nurse consultant, Tina the team administrator and me.

"I know you must be busy but I'd like you to be there," he said

"Brian, I really admire your willingness to have a go, to experiment, take a chance. It's a great example you're setting. I'll be there."

I noticed how his gesture had left me feeling appreciated; such a contrast to some of the responses elsewhere. I gave a good deal of thought to how to be involved. I knew I must resist any temptation to slip into the role of leading these meetings. Instead, I adopted a coaching style: being curious and attentive, asking questions and trying to promote learning. I often felt delighted to be part of these meetings. It enabled me to remain in touch with local, frontline, real-time improvement work, and learn more for myself about how similar QI learning, experience and insights might be shared more widely with other parts of the organisation. I felt inspired by the sense of purpose that seemed so lacking elsewhere. Here this group were doing good work, I felt, that was making a difference to patients.

Although I brought a theoretical knowledge of TOC, I did not insist on the team using this approach. I saw myself as proposing meaning rather than insisting, shaping more than dictating, and offering encouragement. I tried to make sense of some of the challenges we come across using TOC as a paradigm. I go on to describe how I used this approach to contribute to the discussion amongst a group who shared an ambition for improvement.

Fast forward three months and we met again. Brian was chairing. There were two of us in the room and a telephone on a coffee table between us. We heard some distant crackling, "Yes, I can hear you." We knew one another now.

The ward had been operating at 120 percent occupancy for at least the past nine months. The project team worked with the ward's nursing team and developed the idea of a PDDD, the "Patient Determined Discharge Date". This was determined for each patient at the first ward meeting after admission during a discussion between the ward consultant and the patient, with the family present too wherever possible. The ward round had been moved to a meeting room where there was enough wall space to accommodate a large whiteboard, and this now listed all patients by name and incorporated a traffic light system, identifying not only the PDDD but also the date preceding this when that patient's discharge plan needed to be reviewed and if necessary accelerated. The colour coding made those patients approaching their discharge date immediately obvious, and helped focus the team's attention and energies on ensuring everything possible was done to honour this date. At this meeting, I had heard about a discharge coordinator role that had been created for one of the Band 6 nurses. She had been allowed to give up some of her training responsibilities to other colleagues, so that she could focus attention at the ward round on discussions about patients' approaching discharge, and then take a lead thereafter in making sure the discharge plan came together on time. Again I can remember the meeting vividly...

> I summarise what I am hearing, linking this back to TOC. "So I'm hearing you describe small changes, innovations and experiments that you've introduced. Your hunch is it's making a difference in terms of making decisions to prioritise the bottleneck; other work is becoming subordinate to achieving the PDDD."
>
> Then I'm curious: "I'm wondering how you know the effect this is having? Your instinct that it's been useful counts for a lot. But are you also measuring anything that can lend more support to your hunch?"

"Good point." Brian waves a finger while he makes note. "We don't have a data manager. I can tell you we have five outliers, because they're listed in the nursing station. So, just under 120 percent occupancy this week. The IT system is useless, as we all know. So the short answer is no, we're not really measuring anything at the moment."

The administrator speaks for the first time, "The clinical information system won't be able to give you those numbers, but there's new business intelligence software; I went to the training last week. It should be able to give you local, I mean ward level, length of stay and bed occupancy data. I'll look into it and update you at the next meeting."

Everyone seems pleased with this suggestion, and Brian moves on to the next part of the agenda. I am delighted to see such a range of people coming forward with observations and suggestions. This is the inclusivity and creativity I'd hoped for. This work is acquiring a momentum all of its own.

Not so in my more strategic work, which felt more than ever like wading through treacle. My view at the time was that the relationships between the three of us co-leading in our trio and the divisional management teams were vital to the success of all these quality improvement efforts. They would create the conditions in which QI could flourish. If they stayed broken and antagonistic, I feared the flame of local enthusiasm would flicker and die. At this senior level, people were busy, the division large, distances great, and we rarely even caught sight of one another. The agenda of the once-monthly divisional board meeting was overwhelmed with competing and complex issues. Aside from this, with increasing regularity, other meetings were constantly being set up and cancelled at short notice. I was beginning to hear about significant decisions being made at meetings to which I had not been invited. My emails to Pamela, Dave and other senior colleagues often received no response. I began to wonder if there was any method in what felt like a form of madness.

"Am I being intentionally undermined?" I wondered. "Or are we all trying to make the best of a bad deal in whatever we can?" I was finding it increasingly hard to tell.

One afternoon, I bumped into Bob, an old colleague in the HQ building, and he asked me how I am getting on. I crossed my eyes and laughed. He encouraged me to sit down, have a coffee and chat. I told him about what had been going on in the divisional team and about Pamela.

"You can't seriously be telling me all this and then say she's not trying to undermine you! Once, and you can say it's a cock-up, but twice and then a third time? You need to be careful. Are you counting cock-ups or ignoring a conspiracy? You're too patient. She's too complicated," he said, turning his empty paper cup in his hand.

I said, "I can see what you're getting at but I don't think it's as straightforward as that. She can be supportive. In a lot of ways, I quite like her." I noticed I was feeling defensive and attacked.

He said, "She isn't building a team. She isn't using you, your skills. She can't cope with the fact that you're good at what you do. Of course she's undermining you." He gripped the lip of the cup on either side, squashed them together, and then continued to twirl it around.

"As far as I can see, there are competing pressures on her and I suspect she's getting mixed messages too," I said, noticing my feeling of self-control.

"Now I feel like I'm fighting with you! And I'm trying to help you. You're impossible!" he said, crushing the cup and lobbing it into the bin nearby.

I left the conversation not knowing what I had wanted to say. Was this yet another enactment of the drama triangle? Bob tries to rescue me and by appearing to resist his efforts I then become a persecutor to his victim? Is this the drama triangle's cycle repeating itself, its polluting effect threatening now to encroach still further? I was not sure but what proved really helpful about this encounter was that it shone a new light onto a blind spot. Through this open discussion with a trusted friend, I could now see something of my own contribution to the friction and fracture that was arising in the confusion and uncertainty of "joint accountability".

Although I felt as if I was finally beginning to gain some clarity, I began to worry that this muddle and confusing reactivity was becoming increasingly pervasive. I felt alarmed by the sense of derailment I noticed at the start of the next Buttercup Ward project meeting.

> "So they've asked me to move. This is my last meeting," Brian announces unexpectedly.
>
> "But things are just beginning to settle down. It feels like we're really getting somewhere. Do you want to go?"
>
> "I can't say no, can I? I mean, I'm being asked, but I'm being told, aren't I? They've got themselves spooked thinking about the next inspection; they want people going into the eastern sector to embed some systems ASAP."
>
> "But what about the systems we've just got going here?"
>
> After the upbeat meeting of the month before, Parmjeet's arms are folded, her legs are crossed, her head turned half away. "Basically, the

council just doesn't have enough places anyway." She drifts into a pensive silence, and after a minute or two she mutters nonchalantly, "It's not our work anyway. It's the community team's job. And they never show up. Once they get someone admitted then that's it, they bugger off, forget all about them. Out of sight out of mind."

I notice how the focus of the discussion is drifting towards looking at other bottlenecks and how both of these — the council, the community team — are well beyond the project team's sphere of direct influence. I try to name this and begin a discussion on more manageable goals.

"By the way, Tina's off sick. Won't be back for at least three weeks," comes the response.

The tone of this discussion feels much, much flatter. We fall silent. I reflect that this part of my role, supporting quality improvement, has been about asking questions, drawing attention back to what is working, encouraging the team's focus on bottlenecks within their sphere of influence, bringing what influence I can to prevent them becoming weighed down with talking about insoluble problems. In doing so, I have been drawing on Appreciative Inquiry. Using an appreciative approach, I have tried to magnify hopefulness and energy, and offer encouragement. I hope this has done them good and I know it has had a good effect on me. Then something occurs to me, a thought pops into my head, and in the asking and the response we all catch a glimpse of a simultaneous and contrasting reality!

"Brian, how many empty beds have you got today?"

"Five." he says.

"Five?" I say.

"So we're talking about 85 percent occupancy, or thereabouts?" I look at them, my eyes wide open in surprise. They all look back and we begin to chuckle.

"Yes, it's been like that for, well now, what is it, about the last four weeks."

The end

As leaders we strive to generate a sense of common purpose and unity around us, a sense of a good story. I discovered that in the midst of turbulence, transition and change it can be hard to capture the thread of such a story, because it is mostly contrast, change and diversity that make up the raw material of organisational life. However, in the initially rudderless but receptive conditions of the City Services, enthusiasm, dynamism and spontaneity enabled practical improvement solutions to be identified, explored and expanded upon. I felt fortunate that my hope to discover an untapped creativity in frontline settings like Buttercup Ward, to meet local innovators like Brian and Parmjeet, and to become part of a widespread willingness to learn and improve in frontline settings was realised here.

I was surprised at the pace at which those who engaged with QI events, projects and forums embraced Theory of Constraints. I found the Dice Game, and the underlying principles of the theory, easily explained and quickly grasped. With an apparent simplicity that defies the theory's real sophistication, the underlying philosophy, concerned as it is with shared purpose and working effectively together in the interests of the patient, appeared to be welcomed. The basic measurement framework, defining and reducing the length of time that any patient remains in the care system, was widely understood and supported.

On the other hand, and simultaneously, in the confused and confusing strategic corridors of Wilderness Health, good intentions had become constrained by the hidden script of the drama triangle, powerful and deadly, fuelled as it is by unnamed frustration, conflict and fracture. In these circumstances, shared work underpinned by a sense of a common purpose became fatally constrained. This triangle is constructed as a game in which there are three players: victim, persecutor and rescuer. Crucially, as I eventually discovered, the fourth role sitting outside the triangle is concerned with *not* playing the game. Eventually, I came to more fully occupy this position, a place of curiosity, integrity and reflexivity. As I did, I began to explore new leadership gestures inviting different responses, actively inquiring into the rhetoric of "joint accountability" by framing new, open and generous questions. What are the benefits of a system of joint accountability as it stands, and what risks do we run of developing a system of accountability that offers something clearer? What could I do as a leader in this organisation to make myself more accountable to you? What would you need to do to appear more accountable to those you work with? Gradually, the confusion was being untangled and conversations were changing.

What I went on to discover through these questions is the beginning of another story. So, how does this story end? Well, I never did discover if the divisional trio – Pamela, Dave and myself – had been the subject of a covert experiment in implementing complexity thinking. I do know that within a year, each one of us had left our positions and moved on. So for all the successes in the City Services in our work to use TOC to improve quality, I do not know for sure whether my colleagues' improvement work there ultimately won through or was, as I had begun to fear, eventually subsumed by drama. However, in applying the Theory of Constraints as we did, I learnt that our interdependencies in organisational work impose constraints as much as unleash creativity. We set out to create systems that will optimise the latter by moderating the former. Reflection is the tool that provides us with the leverage to work with both.

Engaging
Attracting and
working with others

In Section 2, we saw that having a well-stocked "toolkit" was an advantage when setting out to improve quality, but that on its own, it was insufficient in really getting things moving. A good understanding of Lean or the IHI Method for Improvement or the Theory of Constraints gave some of our contributors the confidence, and indeed the self-belief, to take the first tentative and experimental steps in getting improvement off the ground.

But we also saw that often these first moves hit stony ground. They were rejected or ignored by peers and colleagues and by those who our contributors needed to own the work and make the improvements. Often what was required was some really good relational work (getting to know people better, careful listening, understanding) and some self-examination and re-thinking of an approach which had often been developed in isolation.

In this section, our contributors have found themselves in a context where they feel they want to have a broader scope to their improvement work. One of the contributors was looking to introduce Lean to a mental health service, others were seeking to broaden organisational capability by setting up quality academies in their contexts.

If Section 2 was about beginning and getting things started, the stories in Section 3 offer us some insight into continuing, and getting things moving on a slightly larger scale.

The stories show that there are often surprises and wrong turns. Frequently there is awkwardness, embarrassment, some tears, some joy, but never a smooth path. By staying with their intent, and by being open to emergence and learning, our contributors manage to somehow organise the messiness into something very special.

One story explicitly deals with the subject of power, but power as a theme is bubbling away just below the surface of all of the stories. Making improvement in health needs to be a social act, and our contributors realise this instinctively. They cannot make the difference they want to make alone. And so, they have to work out how best to recruit others, how to engage with other people who may well have different agendas and levels of busy-ness and commitment to improvement. How then, these stories seem to ask, am I to get others to follow me, to work with me, to bring their discretionary effort to this task?

In all the stories the Fellows bring their shifting sense of power to the situation. Not necessarily power in the hierarchical, authoritarian sense, rather as power in the relational "doing with" rather than "doing to" others, in the sense of lighting a flame in others that encourages and enables them to work on the improvement. Finding and accepting this kind of power is often not straightforward, as it is easy to become caught up in our own thoughts, and see the world from too narrow a perspective which doesn't tend to lead to high levels of engagement. In the end, the stories share a similar thread. While our contributors would be the first to say that the journey has only just begun, they all find some way of recognising and using their own power effectively, and learn a great deal about themselves along the way.

There are four stories in this section.
- *Reframing and Seeing the World Differently*, is the story of a surgeon leading a large improvement effort and learning through failure, as well as success, and becoming a more authentic leader in the process
- The second, *Riding the Waves,* is about trying to set up a quality academy in a Trust. There are many twists and turns, some helpful and some less so, with learning about self, others, and the need to get the timing of moves just right
- The third story, *Leaning Out and Letting Go*, is an account of trying to introduce Lean to a mental health service. The Fellow's initial instinct is to use positional power to tell people what to do, but this quickly shifts into realisations around vulnerability and human connection
- The fourth, *Joining the Pack,* is the story of a clinician setting up an

improvement academy who learns how to broker support, confronts his own personal demons, and discovers the joy of leading collaboratively

These stories continue to explore the contextual, relational and personal skills and approaches needed beyond the toolkit. They also suggest that understanding ourselves is an essential prerequisite for engaging with others.

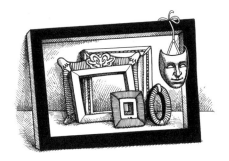

CHAPTER 8

Reframing and Seeing the World Differently

"There weren't enough sweets in the bag for all my friends," said my six-year-old daughter who I'd picked up from school on her birthday.

In her primary school, tradition has it that the birthday boy or girl should give out sweets to their class mates as a celebration, and little did I know that the bag of Haribo I hastily bought at the petrol station that morning only contained 25 sweets. As it turned out, there were not enough for all the class.

"I'm sorry. What did you do?" I waited for the answer with a sense of dread. I had failed as a dad. I'd put a mathematically impossible problem with devastating social consequences upon a six-year-old. Did she split the sweets? Pick her favourite friends? Conduct a lottery? Ask three of her friends who would be gracious enough to forego the bounty?

"I didn't want anyone to be upset." I was still doing my calculations in my head as she spoke. You could split the sweets into two making 50 pieces, that way everyone gets a piece.

"So, did you cut them in half?" My girl was clever, that's what she would have done.

"No daddy, that's silly."

"Oh, so you gave them to your favourite friends?" Please no, I thought.

"No daddy, that's silly."

"Then what did you do?" Maybe the teacher had intervened in what amounted to a child's existential crisis: nothing is more important than friends and Haribo.

"There wasn't enough, so we gave it to reception class."

"That was *very* nice of you." She'd just put my solutions to shame.

Many of the problems I have encountered within the NHS have similarities to that of my daughter's predicament. A finite resource that is not enough to go around, whether it be staffing, theatre space, bed space, money or equipment. The mathematical problem is still the same and there's rarely a chance to increase the resource to meet the demand.

When I reflect upon my behaviour as a clinical leader in my early years, many of my solutions to these apparent conundrums were based upon how to make the demand fit into the existing resources by improving efficiency, reducing waste, reducing variation and getting the teams motivated to work harder. It soon became apparent to me that any success I was achieving was short lived, and just to maintain the improvement I was having to work harder and harder. It often felt like trying to keep a wall of sand propped up; I'd hold one part and another part would slip away.

I started thinking about how my daughter approached her problem. I've noticed that children have a remarkable ability to see the world differently to adults. The fundamental difference was in the way that the problem was framed. My aim would have been the fair distribution of sweets: a finite resource distributed evenly. Her goal had nothing to do with the sweets at all; it was to celebrate her birthday without any one classmate being upset. I'd created a problem that didn't exist because I'd failed to see the bigger picture.

On reflection, many of the mistakes I have made and the lessons I have learnt about leading improvement in the NHS can be attributed to failing to see the world beyond "my problems". It is often those people closest to me who have helped me grow as a leader and who have reminded me to see the world differently.

Leaders don't have the solutions

Many years ago, my hospital was not where you wanted to be if you were ever unfortunate enough to break your hip. Our metrics, according to the National Hip Fracture Database, were amongst the worst in the country, and the complaints from patients and their relatives about the fundamentals of care had become so frequent that alarm bells were ringing at the highest levels of the organisation. It was clear we needed urgent change.

I put together the largest multidisciplinary team imaginable and led upon an ambitious project to elevate our quality of care to the best in class and to provide the "right care, in the right place at the right time". Over the course of six months, the whole process of care from the ambulance service, accident and emergency, the wards, operating theatre and post-operative care were remapped, engaging key stakeholders in each group. This project was of such importance – to me at least – that I was never absent in any of the over 100 meetings that were held.

The methodology involved remapping using Lean principles, designing a new pathway, and creating a new clinical bundle of care which I proudly presented nationally as *the* solution to improvement.

As we began implementation of the proposed new pathway, I began to be made aware of problems. Few to start with, and small, and then progressively more and more and bigger. The pathway that we had designed was so idealised and aspirational, so far removed from current reality, that even a person with a cursory understanding of our hospital could tell that it was impossible – if they cared to "go look see". For example, it's impossible to admit a patient from the hospital front door to the ward within two hours when the average wait to obtain a hospital bed at the time was over six hours. It's impossible to operate upon a patient within 24 hours from admission when many patients are still stuck in the accident and emergency department. It's impossible that all patients be reviewed by an orthogeriatrician post-operatively when we didn't even have one.

Each implementation meeting became a list of problems directed at me. After all, I was their designated leader, and one passionate about improving the quality of care. The more problems I had, the harder I worked at trying to find solutions. After 12 months of trying to implement the new pathway, the metrics had not improved, and the complaints had increased.

Why had all this work resulted in apparently no difference? I began to question my ability to lead change, to take people with me, and increasingly became exhausted.

One evening at home, after a particularly late meeting, I developed severe palpitations and felt a sense of dread as I dropped to the floor. I heard my wife shouting at me.

"Why are you doing this to us?" I felt physically sick. Was I having a heart attack? This was the last thing I wanted to hear from her.

"Don't you realise how important the work I do is?" You could at least acknowledge that, I felt myself thinking.

"No, you're not doing it for them, you're doing it for yourself."

It was not until later that her statement sank in. She was right. The reason why I wanted to lead the change was because of pride for my department and to achieve a great improvement. I was also in the grip of my Try Hard driver (see Appendix 3) and I could not bear the thought of failure. Unintentionally, I had succumbed to grandiosity and had created a vision that was unrealistic and, rather than empower the team to share responsibility for the change, I had created dependency. I have since learned that leaders who run too far ahead of their own teams are destined to fail for many reasons. They lose credibility, because the project becomes more about them than the original purpose. Team paralysis sets in, as no action can be taken without the presence of the leader, and when the leader becomes tired any changes will revert to the previous norm. I had experienced all of these and more. I had a lot to learn about both leading complex change and developing my own resilience.

I started to learn that to influence change within my organisation, I had to change first. I had to understand my own motivations for leading change, and I realised how easy it is for hubris to set in. Leadership is not about me, or them, but us. The role of a leader is not to provide a list of solutions to the perceived problems, but to create a conducive culture where improvement problems can be explored, reframed and the bigger picture understood.

I still remember the day that the implementation effort quite suddenly and unexpectedly turned direction, moving away from the pathway- and metric-driven approach which I had chosen. It was the day that I invited six of our previous patients to come to our implementation team meeting with their families, including those who had recently complained about their care.

After I had presented the new care pathway to them, focusing upon all the benefits it would unleash, one of the elderly gentlemen who had recently recovered from his hip fracture stood up to speak. He reminded me of my own family members who have the courage to break the silence and name the elephant, telling it as it is, just as my wife had done for me when I was on the point of collapse.

"This is all very impressive, but I honestly don't care about any of this stuff. I don't know any of this medical jargon. What I care about is the fact that you didn't tell me anything when I came into hospital and no one seemed to listen when I had a problem. We all trust you'll do the surgery right, but it's the other things which are important to me."

It seems so obvious now, but at the time it was both a relief and a revelation. We had spent so much time and effort trying to solve intractable and complex problems, and here was a patient telling us that talking and listening were the most important things, and that he trusted us to get the rest right. Talking and listening; we must be able to do that with no additional cost, no extra resource, no extra effort. Surely?

This was the start of the reframing of our work, from a hip fracture pathway redesign to providing a patient- and family-centred model of care. I was able to engage the team to remap the patient journey, considering all aspects of care from the eyes of the patient, and focus effort upon those areas which patients cared about the most. I have since learned that in making this shift I was using some of the principles of another approach, Experience Based Co-design (EBCD).

The most illuminating and rewarding aspect of this shift was what happened to our pathway metrics, which we had failed to improve in the first 12 months. They spontaneously started improving without any extra effort or changes to the pathway. How could the time to surgery improve by 40% in a six-month period when *apparently* nothing had changed?

I learnt that change occurs when we believe in what we are doing and in who we are doing it for, when everyone takes charge to make things better. It was no longer about me, or an idealised future state.

Don't be the hero

I learned a lot about leading change from the hip pathway improvement project. I also learned a great deal about my impact on key relationships, and how, with good intent, I can undermine the very people I greatly valued. Through the project, I nearly lost relationship with Ann, a very senior nurse who I worked closely with, and who I valued and admired enormously.

As well as the poor outcome metrics, the complaints we were receiving before the start of the project were very serious, and accountability for them fell upon Ann's shoulders. One evening, following a long day of operating, I received a call from the nursing director saying that Ann was to be suspended due to a lack of leadership on her part, resulting in failings of care. Of all the nurses I had met in my life, Ann was the most compassionate, dedicated and gentle human being I knew. I felt angry that the organisation had chosen to scapegoat, in my view, such a dedicated individual.

"This is totally unjust, I can't believe you are thinking about suspending one of the most brilliant nurses I know." I protested her innocence.

I couldn't sit back and just let this happen to someone I trusted and believed in. Something had to be done. I phoned the Nursing Director the following day and proposed that Ann and I would embark on a quality improvement project together, and that within 12 months our quality of care would be dramatically better. In my mind, I wanted to save her because she didn't deserve this.

You need to understand the kind of person and nurse she was. Ann was loved by all the ward staff. They saw her like a mother, and her empathy with patients set an example for everyone else to follow. My regard and concern for Ann was one of the reasons why I'd put my head above the parapet and embarked upon the hip fracture project at all. Looking back, it was probably as important to me as my concern about our clinical outcomes.

As the project got underway I began to sense a change in the relationship between Ann and her staff. Ann seemed more withdrawn and there wasn't the usual buzz of energy amongst her staff in the ward. The mood had shifted, and at the time it was hard to put a finger on what had happened. Looking back now, the shadow of scrutiny was ever present, and people knew that Ann was being judged and was at risk. I can also see that I had effectively taken over the lead for quality on the ward, and in doing so I had unwittingly pushed Ann aside. I had unleashed the Karpman drama triangle (Karpman 2011) where acting as the rescuer, the hero, I had unwittingly cast Ann as the victim and disempowered her.

Eventually, Ann left the ward to move to another, leaving behind her staff who she had cared for so much and who had respected her in return.

"I wish you had never made that phone call to the director," she said, as our parting goodbye. At that moment, I was the victim, persecuted by the very person I had set out to rescue.

As I reflect now I can very easily berate myself for how I treated Ann, and yet I can also see that it is only natural that most of us in health care want to help people. We are altruistic by our very nature. And yet, the way we go about offering this help can lead to unintended consequences. When I view the NHS, I can see a great institution trying, perhaps unintentionally, to be the hero of society; saving patients from the persecution of disease. I fear that the more the NHS behaves as the hero, the more patients might become the victims, dependent on the hero to solve their problems. A day might come when the hero can no longer continue saving the victim and, on that day, the victim will turn and persecute the hero. I've learnt that sustainable change within the NHS can only come from working *with* patients and not for them, when responsibility is shared and, using Transactional Analysis terminology (Lapworth and Sills 2011) [see Appendix 2 for more on this], we all behave as Adults.

You'll be glad to hear that Ann returned to the ward after six months and we started our improvement project again. I was so relieved. This time we listened to the values and experiences of patients and their families, and merged them with the metrics we had previously determined. To our surprise, it was the apparently little things that really mattered in their care: empathy, communication, a simple cup of tea, the ability to have a quiet night's sleep. As for all the rest – well – patients trusted us to do our best. Listening to our patients allowed us to reframe the problem and find the simple solutions that my daughter would have found.

The power of purpose

At the time that Ann and I were working together it was traditional for most wards in our hospital to have a raffle for a Christmas hamper, with donations for the hamper made by members of staff. Ticket sales for the hamper would go towards the ward fund to pay for extra equipment, such as a mobile TV or even the Christmas decorations. On Christmas Day that year an eight-year-old boy was visiting his grandfather, who was recovering from a broken hip. Ann knew that the grandfather was particularly fond of his whisky and took a small bottle from the hamper and gave it to him. The boy saw how happy this simple gesture made his grandfather. He also saw all the other elderly patients around him, many without family visiting them on this Christmas evening.

He wanted everyone in hospital at Christmas to receive a gift, as his grandfather had done, and set about collecting money with a sponsored run.

The following year, he came to the same ward on Christmas Eve with sacks of presents, and told the story of why he was there and what he wanted to be done with the presents. He left without giving his name or telling us who his grandfather was. To this day, we have no idea who he is. Perhaps he is reading this story now.

I was on call that day and I received a phone call from Ann who was so excited and moved by what this little boy had done. I too was moved by such a beautiful act of kindness which originated from a simple gesture of empathy from a nurse. I tweeted his inspiring story, just 24 words. *#Realsanta* spread across the organisation, and many more wards started giving out their Christmas hampers to their patients that year.

I reflected upon how a boy, who is only eight years old, could create resonating change across an organisation. When I heard his story, my thinking began to shift in a profound way. Could it be that shifts in behaviour and culture across an organisation occur when staff can *feel* the significance of the change, rather than being persuaded by an objective rationale? Is that why patient stories appear to have had a much greater influence in changing how we work than scientific redesign?

Since then, I have learned about the power of stories in influencing positive change. In my experience, whilst stories do not provide the solutions to the perceived problems, they inspire and enable people within an organisation to change beyond the apparent constraints of the system.

The NHS is not a machine. It is a living breathing entity made up of staff, patients, families and the public, all of whom care. To build upon this analogy, quality improvement keeps the NHS fit and breathing well. It requires regular disciplined training and leaders who lead by example. It is grounded in the here and now, and it requires people to *feel* the need for change, and for leaders to inspire those around them at an emotional level.

I believe as leaders we must ask ourselves what motivates us to do what we do. I thought I was the type of leader to lead by example, and had the skills to achieve great improvements. I have learned that in the early days I did what I did because I wanted to be *seen* to achieve great improvements. What I now do is no longer about me or them. It is about us. Change can rarely be attributed to any one person, and always happens through conversations where meaning and a shared purpose can emerge.

And, just occasionally, and often unexpectedly, tectonic shifts can occur.

Are we family?

Since the story I have just shared, I have had many moments of feeling proud of what we achieve together in the NHS. One of the best occurred as I listened to a seminal lecture given by a surgeon I had trained many years previously. His research was beautifully planned and executed. The novel surgery he had developed and validated through his research was something that I had just started to learn myself, and here was a young consultant surgeon who had already surpassed my experience and contribution in such a short time. I was simultaneously both proud and jealous of him.

During the coffee break he asked to speak with me privately, so we sat down in a quiet corner. I half expected him to ask for career advice or feedback on his lecture.

"I just wanted to say that, if it wasn't for you, I wouldn't be where I am now. You started it all for me."

In that moment, I felt profound pride as a father might, such as the time my daughter was able to play *Für Elise* better than I could remember from my teenage years. It made me think about how I view my colleagues, other staff members, the trainee surgeons assigned to me, and my patients. Were they just good people I work with, or were they more than that? What would the impact be upon the culture of health care if we were able to change and reframe the way we perceive the people around us, if we were able to reframe the way we perceive ourselves?

In my current role I am often invited to give a talk. On many occasions, before I start, I ask the audience to describe the stereotypical orthopaedic surgeon. The responses are sometimes far from flattering: arrogant, workaholic, think they are God's gift, money grabbing, bullies – these are some of the more temperate comments. It's not for me to defend my profession because I do see all those things. Nevertheless, I have the privilege of seeing who my colleagues *are*, and not just how they sometimes behave.

As a leader, I used to feel that I should behave as I believed a leader should: out there in front, strong, with a vision and in control. Every morning I would put on a mask so that I could lead by example. I would be careful about what I said for fear of expressing an opinion that would be wrongly construed. I feared expressing doubt, weakness or showing vulnerability. Ever so slowly I started *feeling* like the leader I thought I should be. I started to become the mask. The more I began to feel like the leader wearing the mask – in my work, with my family, in private – I started to behave more and more like the stereotypical orthopaedic surgeon.

I believe that many of us in health care do this – behave as if we are the mask. Maybe it is a way of protecting ourselves from the emotional impact of having to care for patients, of being able to make those surgical incisions, of living with the everyday reality of possible death. Maybe the only way we can conduct our professional duties is if we remain emotionally detached. And yet, if this is "true", it comes at a great cost, to ourselves as human beings and to our patients. The NHS is not a machine, our patients are not cogs in the machine, and nor are our colleagues.

The most powerful and difficult lesson I have learnt through my leadership career is to let go of the mask of leadership and to be who I really am. I've learnt to be that old gentleman who's not afraid of saying just what he thinks, or my daughter who can see the world, not by the measure of sweets, but the emotional wellbeing of the people around her.

It's allowed me to lead, with others, a movement in my profession to try and change the culture of surgery. Shifting culture results in a generational paradigm shift and is not populated by heroes. No longer the arrogant bullies, but a more nurturing, caring and empathetic family of people.

I bet you never thought you would hear an orthopaedic surgeon say that!

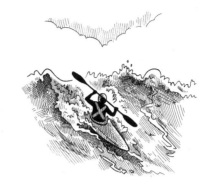

CHAPTER 9

Riding the Waves

It started with a conversation. Most of the significant developments and progress I have observed seem to begin this way. Perhaps it's because of the importance of creating connections rather than just developing abstract plans?

I arranged to meet with the Chief Executive. Of itself this was a change of practice for me. Instead of going through the committee process I wanted to understand his particular view with the aim of developing a common ambition.

I arrived for the meeting mindful of how I needed to project my message, aware I can be animated and enthusiastic and not take time to listen as much as I ought, but also confident I had something important to say. I felt well prepared.

The conversation that followed about the vision for improvement surprised me. The questions I expected to be asked did not materialise, and instead I was asked "When can you make this happen?"

I had become so used to not making progress, and to having to defend proposals, that the unexpected question surprised me so much I completely forgot to negotiate any commitment to the resources or support I might need! However, looking back, it was this meeting that sparked the beginning of the Academy. I now needed to work on creating a groundswell of opinion that would support this becoming our strategic approach to improvement.

But I have done what I always do – allowed my enthusiasm to begin to take over. Let me give you some background first....

Background

In 2015, I set out with the ambition to have a lasting impact on the culture of our organisation, to try to create the conditions to support quality improvement which would enable our staff to move beyond the rhetoric of improvement to its actual delivery. The idea was to challenge, inspire and empower all the people of our organisation to consider what they might do better, and with skill and support bring about change for good in their everyday work.

At the same time, I wanted to create a system which provided focus and direction for structured quality improvement (QI) to take place at scale. In short, I wanted a Quality Academy and the ambition within the hospital to support QI, improve patient care, develop capability in our staff and make it a better place to be. I wanted these changes to be sustained in the long term.

I had spent time thinking through how the Academy might work and identified the groups that would need to be involved and the importance of certain individuals to the progress of my ideas. For the meeting with the Chief Executive I had prepared a short visual presentation (avoiding death by PowerPoint!), hoping it would keep our conversation focused given the short time available. I chose not to address the governance, accountability and delivery structures that might need to sit around my proposal, as with so much uncertainty, nailing down specifics was going to be hard and might fix our direction too soon, rather than allowing it to emerge. The approach proved to have merits, both in the meeting and the subsequent work.

Uncertainty becomes the norm

I am mindful as I write that it is all too easy to portray this story as if it followed a narrative I had predetermined, but it didn't. I did have a plan, but everyday crises, changes of opinion, changes of staff, financial uncertainty, regulator pressure and new ideas – including good ones – continually seemed to batter progress. Sometimes, feelings of aloneness and isolation as well as frustration had to be dealt with. Even now I still carry the feeling that at any moment the carpet might be dragged unceremoniously from under the considerable progress that has been made, and I still wonder what would happen were I taken out of the equation. Is our organisation's commitment to quality improvement still based on the enthusiasm and drive of so few that it remains precarious to the pressures of productivity and the need to make the books balance?

Such uncertainty, paradoxically, appears to be one of the most certain features of my experience, and I have had to learn to deal with it and not let it overwhelm me. As a leader for quality improvement I have become increasingly aware of the significance and disruptive influence of life's uncertainties and ambiguities on my work and ambitions, as well as their impact on my patients and the colleagues with whom I work. The problem of course is that, "life happens". As I write these opening paragraphs I am painfully aware that just a week ago my partner and I sat in the kitchen while I shaved her head, AC/DC playing at full tilt in the background, as we both cried. She is just finishing her first cycle of chemotherapy and managing a little better than we expected. But there's a long road to go.

Over these past few months our experience of health care has been mixed, some of it good, some of it bad. Working in the same hospital in which she is being treated has given us the privilege of experiencing friends and colleagues looking after us with kindness and dignity, whilst at the same time we have been frustrated by the inefficiencies of the system within which we work. It is probably an experience common to many of our patients.

Whilst this experience has confirmed my belief in the essential requirement of quality improvement to be an integral part of the way we develop health care, it has also demonstrated, all too clearly, the way that the random events of everyday work and life sometimes derail the smooth execution of our plans.

For our patients, hope and love are what seem to be required to deal with the situations they face. Hope created by their experience of the care they receive, despite the uncertainties of their situation. Trust and confidence, strengthened by their encounters of well-delivered safe, effective and efficient care built around their needs. And, when that is just not possible, because of the finality of their condition, love. Compassionate care which recognises their needs and aspirations, and which enables them to deal with their pain and fear. Care which draws alongside them in a supportive and comforting way.

At the same time, I believe it is important that we, as improvers, are also helped to be able to deal with the impact of the uncertainties of organisational and personal life on us and our work. Developing such capacity has built my resilience. It has also made work more enjoyable and sustainable, as it provides hope that what I am trying to achieve is possible, despite the ever-changing environment and the uncertainties we face when trying to sustain a competent and capable health service.

Understanding myself

So for better or worse, I had negotiated for myself a mandate to get on and set up a Quality Academy. My passion and motivation were off the scale. My motivation for the Academy and for quality improvement grew from observing the experience of our patients. I had been struck by their disarming joy at their expectations of care frequently being surpassed; but on other occasions I had been distressed by their disappointment, frustrations and even anger with ineffective and unreliable systems that led to delays, uncertainty, anxiety and harm.

That the latter experience happens all too frequently fuelled my passion and energy to try to shape the system, to enable our staff to provide the care they really wanted to. However, the darker side of such motivation is that it also fuels potentially disruptive personal frustration and sometimes anger at lack of progress in making such change. Emotions that, when harnessed, are useful, but unfettered resulted in loss of perspective and context, reducing my capacity for constructive debate. Learning to achieve a balance between these reactions has allowed me to step back and to take a more considered view. Not losing my passion, but balancing it with an appreciation of the bigger picture.

I remember many occasions where this passion would boil over into frustration. My interactions with senior management had resulted on occasion in me being perceived as reactive, emotional, and unable to see the bigger context. I remember being asked whether I was "tired out" when energetically detailing failings of care for some of our patients. The risk was that I was making myself feel better (sometimes) but changing little.

On reflection, I realised that my instinctive reaction, that of emotional outrage, was not enough.

I had to learn to behave differently; to understand more about my instinctive reactions. Instead of reacting in the same old way, I needed to take time to listen and develop an idea or a viewpoint by holding it up to others for scrutiny and comment, enabling a generative way of conversing where different views are shared. To my relief, this also reduced my personal stress, as I no longer needed to fight my corner. Instead I embraced others' views which led to better outcomes than I would have achieved alone.

For instance, two sets of colleagues were fighting over the safest way to deliver a particular aspect of care. Instead of making a snap decision, I took time to reflect and appreciate their relative positions. Instead of negotiating a compromise, I took the time to visit the unit, where I came to understand more fully the impact of difficult events that had led to their disagreement by listening to staff and patients who had been affected by organisational changes to a surgical pathway. This change of perspective and approach meant that rather than becoming exasperated at two seemingly intractable positions, I was able to bring the two sides closer together by understanding and reframing their viewpoints, which was sufficient to bring about a collaborative solution rather than a contrived and unsatisfactory compromise. Understanding myself better, my inclination to jump to solutions, provided me with an improved "depth" perspective when tackling difficult improvement issues. In a similar way, it allowed me to articulate more clearly the case for the Academy in a constructive and inclusive manner, by taking time to understand my senior colleagues' viewpoints and concerns.

The waves begin

Following the initial enthusiasm and progress we had made with developing the ideas for QI in the hospital, I began to face the fact that little was happening. Even with my more considered approach, I found engaging with the executive difficult. They were busy and already had their agenda filled by our financial issues and the constant need to meet regulator demands. In the same way, our frontline staff who recognised the need for improvement seemed constrained by a lack of time and the demands of their everyday jobs.

This created a number of unwanted consequences. I became frustrated, those involved in projects started to disappear, and the executive started to question what progress was being made.

Slowly but surely the impetus seemed to be ebbing away.

I decided to take a new tack. It was a risk. I had a reasonable working relationship with a colleague who was part of the senior team who, although sometimes perceived as confrontational, was a strong advocate for QI. Not the style of QI I was accustomed to, but keen for improvement nonetheless. His style could be seen as abrasive, but he had a directness that I felt could be helpful and a place at the top table, together with the skills to make things happen. I decided to meet and share my vision and to spend time listening to his views and approach.

Our meeting was interesting. As I had experienced before, it was difficult to be able to express an alternative viewpoint without raising significant reservations. This escalated to the point where it seemed unlikely he would be an advocate of the Academy. We got so far and then he shut down the conversation. My natural inclination was to defend my position, but I was at the time experimenting with Isaacs' ideas (1999) around developing dialogue and was determined to suspend my view, moving away from advocacy to inquiry, listening as carefully as I could to what he had to say, properly allowing him to express his "voice".

When I recounted this story to a colleague, she pointed out that the antagonism and push back I was experiencing was in fact because he was actually engaged and interested. He was occupying one of the four positions described by Isaacs required for dialogue to evolve – the Opposer – constructive disagreement. Initially I had felt defensive, but in working hard to understand his perspective, the conditions to develop a more rounded plan began to emerge.

He later called me, explaining that he had reflected on our conversation. His shutting down of the conversation had in fact been a moment he required for synthesis, rather than a rejection of the ideas I had offered.

His later involvement and support would go on to underpin the Academy moving forward.

Understanding the organisational context

So now, I felt as though I was beginning to make some forward strides in setting up the Academy. I had learned new ways of engaging with people, and had recruited senior team members to keep the momentum going. I felt the need now to try to align the move toward a quality improvement approach with other organisational goals, so that QI would become an essential part of what we did every day.

However, as an Associate Director, I felt I was not always fully inside the inner circle of decision-making and planning for the organisation. It has benefits, as I can focus more on what I need to do in the limited time I have available, but has the downside of making me susceptible to being sideswiped by new projects and ideas or problems facing the executive. I use the term sideswiped as there is a real sensation sometimes of being knocked off balance. I now realise such events are inevitable. Understanding this makes my intentions much more likely to survive the inevitable waves and perturbations.

Knowing that the top team respond particularly well to projects with evidence of success helps me prepare an engaging account, which captures their imagination and fuels ongoing support for the Academy, even in the face of challenges. Just this week I was delighted, and perhaps a little bit shocked, to hear the CEO state that the Quality Academy is now one of our underpinning strategies guiding the work of the hospital. This statement was made to a visiting Government Minister and the Great and Good of the hospital.

> *Personal reflections? I am amused to reflect that despite this demonstration of senior commitment, instead of unbridled joy, I felt an increased burden of responsibility. A surprise, as I always viewed myself as an optimist. This fits with the personal expectations which writers such as Binney (2012) say leaders are sometimes burdened with, and underlines the importance of distributed leadership.*
>
> *This is something I repeatedly need to manage with care as it would be unhealthy if the Academy was perceived by the executive or by me as my sole responsibility. Such a responsibility would likely weaken it, increasing the likelihood of failure, and make it personally draining and arduous.*

To protect the Academy (and myself), the Academy needed to be about more than me or short-term relationships. To ground our expectations, I arranged a series of meetings with the executive, examining how we incorporate our quality ambitions more closely with the everyday work of the hospital. It seemed essential to link QI to the operational effectiveness of the hospital, in addition to the safety work of the organisation which, so far, had been our principal focus. They were challenging conversations, as it was necessary to address the constraints of developing understanding and acceptance of QI, acknowledging the needs of patients to be met, and the requirements imposed by external regulators, whose target-driven approach sometimes distorts priorities.

Dealing with such meetings and conversations has required me to develop a better understanding of the use of power and politics; in this context using what has been described by Wiggins (2016) as soft power, "The ability to get others to think the way you do".

To be able to use such power effectively required me to understand how the senior team operates. To have any influence required the support of key decision makers. Without this I have discovered that my plans rarely have any longevity or sustainability. I have learned that constantly refreshing support for the QI strategy helps the senior team, both to offer them assurance, but more importantly to provide them with the opportunity to become intimately involved. Meeting individually with the executive, listening to their views and eliciting their concerns and ideas armed with a clear message and an aim articulated in diagram, pictures, written words and presentations helped hugely.

Each time I did this it helped bring individuals on board, sparking new themes for collaboration, and enabling them to take steps to support our next steps. This was particularly beneficial with the HR and OD teams, who agreed that quality improvement would be discussed in all staff appraisals, that all new staff would have an induction which would feature QI as an expectation of hospital life, and that recruitment would include QI as a value for which we positively select.

I also tried to link national strategy to our local plans to promote our QI work. For instance, outlining how the financial and operational benefits of reducing length of stay for patients with respiratory issues would help meet the external targets placed on the executive. For example, within our grasp was the potential of releasing more than five-hundred bed days a year, improved outcomes for patients, and reduced costs of patient care. For the Quality Academy it demonstrated the importance of having capable teams who are conversant in QI methodology.

Understanding and making the most of complexity

Surfing the waves

The story so far has been *lumpy*, a kayaker's term for an unpredictable sea, and I am a keen kayaker. Negotiating lumpiness has been both testing and exciting. Throughout the development of the Academy this metaphor has proved helpful. When I started as Associate Director I was aware that getting things done in my hospital was complicated. It frequently required lots of energy and time to sustain any changes that were achieved. However, at that point I had failed to fully appreciate the impact of complexity.

Early in my experience of trying to set up the Academy, I had assumed that commitment and energy combined with force of will alongside the development of strategic alliances would be the key determinants of success. This approach helped, but what I hadn't fully appreciated was the impact of the randomness and chaos of the everyday, the lumpy sea, that required an ability to ride the waves or the wind sometimes in unexpected directions.

The impact on me has been significant. No plan seems to progress in a straight line without the need for continuous refinement and adaptability. It makes work tiring and demands a lot of time keeping things on track.

Stacey and other authors describe the concept of complexity and its relevance to organisational change well [see Appendix 1], challenging the very notion of organisations as entities, proposing instead that organisations consist of patterns of individuals interacting with each other. Such a way of looking at organisations has proved valuable and reassuring; legitimising my experience. When formulating strategy, it has helped me realise that planning to get from A to C is not simply a matter of going through B in a straight line. All manner of individual behaviours, interactions and conditions serve to upset that level of simplistic thinking.

Until I accepted this reality – *really* accepted it – I was becoming increasingly frustrated. Frustrated because plans for the Academy were so often changed or buffeted by uncertainty that it seemed nothing would ever succeed. As Stacey suggests, "What happens in an organisation is not simply the consequence of choices made by powerful people... instead it is the interplay between the many choices and actions of all involved." (2012, p. 4)

For this reason, it became increasingly important to try to influence the context in which the individuals working in our hospital operated, whilst at the same time working opportunistically; accepting that leading and managing a programme of work like this will rarely deliver as anticipated, but will most likely require continuous nudging and cajoling to get somewhere close to the perceived objective. Even a simple matter such as creating a video to support a new induction process required flexibility on our part, the expected resource not being available, agreement needing to be negotiated. However, staff from a completely unexpected team were able to step up. In the process we created new alliances as well as great videos that have subsequently proved very successful.

Setting the rhythm for improvement

I found it particularly helpful to have created appropriate structures to support quality improvement. A key step was to separate quality assurance processes from quality improvement. This has been particularly instrumental in moving QI up the ladder of importance in the Trust's priorities as, until that point, quality assurance had dominated the quality agenda, improvement being the "poor relation".

By focusing on investigating individual problems we were failing to consistently deliver improvement work. We knew what was wrong, but were spending too little time improving. Once the two were separated (we now have a committee for each), we were more able to prioritise improvement work streams and set up and observe their metrics. In this way, we were able to develop a top ten of organisational improvement objectives, and to consider other aspects of improvement work, such as resourcing and capability development, through the Quality Academy. This has led to specific QI programmes achieving measurable improvement.

Working on consistency while avoiding turf wars

Whilst developing the Academy and broadening its membership, we brought together a range of individuals and teams with their associated expertise from around the hospital. This diversity increased the reach of the Academy, propelling it forwards, but it also brought with it some challenges. In particular, we experienced the need to maintain cohesiveness and consistency in approach, which on occasion required adaptation of focus and working practices as we struggled to secure a more common purpose. For instance, our human factors team have been persuaded to examine how they might extend their current training programmes to address organisational goals in line with our overarching QI objectives. Developing a conjoined driver diagram is helping us work through this collaboratively.

At the same time, it was important to recognise the potential for such changes to cause a perceived loss of autonomy and erosion of power and influence.

Recognising the leadership and responsibilities of others in their improvement work has been critical. In the past, I was guilty of taking on work which others should have completed. This led to me becoming overloaded and overwhelmed at times. Being able to let go of personal responsibility required me to relinquish control whilst still being able to call the general direction; to be "in charge but not in control".

Take for instance our sepsis programme. We used to meet regularly to discuss the progress we were making in all areas in a sepsis improvement group. Due to the increasing operational pressures in our emergency department and issues of flow through the hospital, we found that fewer and fewer were able or willing to attend the meeting due to other commitments.

The risk was that, as lead for the programme, I would work around this by collecting their data for them and taking on some of their responsibility. On occasion, this was appropriate, but in the long term unsustainable. The solution was to intermittently cancel the central meeting and instead go to the local areas where the issues were emerging. This allowed area-specific work plans to be co-designed, and provided the opportunity to see work in practice rather than work as described. It felt more creative, and improved local buy-in and relationships. In the long term, I hope it will also lead to greater autonomy and ownership of their improvement plans. It does mean I have more meetings to go to, but they are much shorter and more relevant, I don't waste others' time, and it is a joy to see others stepping up to take responsibility. Some of the tasks, I relinquished altogether.

Working more opportunistically

As I look back now I can see that the trail taken moving forwards with our improvement agenda is littered with opportunistic events. Fires lit, through occasional but frequent conversations with all kinds of staff along the way, only later truly blazed into life and created new and unexpected opportunities.

I have learned that my most successful projects were those where I formed alliances with others. For instance, at the outset of pitching for the Academy I constructed a stakeholder plan, and conducted a sustained programme of meetings with all my stakeholders to gauge their opinions and garner support. I found an "elevator pitch" for each meeting to be helpful, describing clearly the concept of the Quality Academy. During these meetings I listened, relaxing my need for pre-determined outcome, recognising that others might have views of what the Academy might be. Dialogue provided space for such uncertainty, and I was delighted by the creativity that resulted. As a consequence, the inception of the Academy came as much from stakeholders as from me, and they became active participants.

Taking the time to have opportunistic and unplanned "corridor" conversations also helped create alliances, which later provided the momentum for progress when individuals who later came together in "formal" meetings had already engaged in similar conversations. True back-stage and front-stage political work. Eventually, I hope I will no longer need to be present to advocate for the Academy, as there will be a developing collective leadership.

As an example, following an opportunistic pilot training course, I was talking to a group of enthusiastic colleagues and we all decided that it would be great to run a new course entitled "QI for dummies". The idea seemed to land very well. This year we have increased our participants from 12 to 28 medical students, each helping to lead QI initiatives. The opportunities created for these students is now starting to open up the possibility of a medical undergraduate course in QI, human factors and leadership as part of the Academy portfolio.

Change and be changed

To successfully lead change, I have had to change. At times, it has been an uncomfortable process. Much of this change was facilitated through my GenerationQ programme of study, and through the considered support and feedback of my friends on the programme.

Perhaps the most valuable skill I have learned was developing my reflective practice. This has increased my resilience, broadened my understanding of myself, and increased my thinking horizon hugely. Learning through reflection has been the process which has helped me guide and develop how I work, rather than just acting instinctively. I have come to understand that I have an inclination to *Please Others* [see Appendix 3]. This has helped me realise why sometimes progress with ideas seemed slow. In discussion with the senior team they articulated that they sometimes felt that I waited for permission or approval to get on with projects. In part this related to the culture, which I felt required such an approach, but undoubtedly part of the issue rested with me and my choice of behaviours. So now I try to be ten percent braver, take the risk and get on with it. It is rarely a bad experience, although it does occasionally catch people by surprise, so a bit of signposting of this change in behaviour can be helpful!

The impact of this approach in general has been effective. Understanding better my leadership style made it easier for me to develop strategic alliances with the HR and OD departments of the hospital, as well as with the service improvement teams. This in turn has had significant influence on the impetus of the QI programme, as it has become much more a shared endeavour. It has started to generate the conditions for a system wide approach to QI with a common goal and greater synergy between different parts of the organisation. This in turn is creating opportunities of scale, which I hope will help unlock some of the resources required to support our staff to develop QI capabilities.

Hopefully these changes have been good for the projects I lead. They have certainly been good for me. When I listen more carefully, with greater acuity, I find I rush in less, am more considered, and have an increased ability to respond well to others, taking into account the external context. I am also more able to reflect afterwards and notice what is taking place. That doesn't mean I get it right every time. Rushing in seems to have been a specialist area for me, and I need to take care not to return to such instinctive behaviours.

When I take care to respect others and listen it makes me less defensive and reactive. Looking for the best in others and taking responsibility for the impact in my thinking helps stop me jumping to premature or even the wrong conclusions.

I have also learned the benefits of careful signposting and saying clearly what I think. I am developing my own personal culture, an ability to voice the real me and say what I believe whilst remaining open to others' points of view.

Despite many positives there remains considerable uncertainty which I, as an improver, need to deal with. This, coupled with the complexity of working in a large health care organisation, has underlined to me the importance of being able to share my struggles with supportive work colleagues and friends, who have experienced the same frustrations, lack of progress and setbacks. Sharing the good, the bad and the ugly has been really helpful in building my personal resilience, by increasing my under-standing of leadership, better enabling me to deal with complexity and its impact on me more effectively.

Perhaps most importantly, as a consequence of my learning I am happier to be in charge but not in control when the context requires it (Streatfield 2001). This encourages me to defend my position less, so less advocacy and more inquiry. It has provided me with a set of skills that help me deal more comprehensively with the uncertainties of work life and life in general.

Dedicated to the memory of my friend, patient and inspiration, the potter RG, who took simple clay and by some alchemy created the extraordinary.

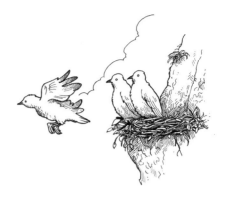

CHAPTER 10

Leaning Out and Letting Go

It was a sunny Thursday morning and my stomach was churning. I sat in the meeting that I had arranged thinking, "Who do I think I am? Who am I to tell these experienced clinicians what they should do?" Then I thought, "You are not trying to tell them what to do. Your intention here is to join with them to think about how to improve services for children and young people. You have some expertise here; it does no one any good to hide that in case people think you're bossy. We are under so much pressure in the NHS, we have to make improvements. This is not about you, this is about those young people having to go far from their homes to get a hospital bed. You know how we can improve flow and reduce waste. Lean in."

Me and my work

I am a consultant psychiatrist working in a children and young people's mental health service. For years I have seen the problems of under investment and unacceptably long waits for our service. Seventy-five percent of all long-term adult mental health problems are apparent by young adulthood. We know the children who are struggling and will become adults who will be significantly impacted by their mental health problems. Nevertheless, we are chronically underfunded and it's yet another example of the stigma around mental health. For example, I met with a 17-year-old girl the other day who had been struggling with symptoms of trauma (flash-backs, nightmares, anxiety, avoidance of situations) since she was 14. She had been on a waiting list to be seen for over 12 months. Her avoidance and anxiety is now so habitual that it's going to be very difficult to get her back into school to complete her A levels. Yet less than one percent of the NHS budget is spent on child and adolescent mental health.

I feel really passionate about young people being able to access care as soon as they need it. One way I thought we could make a difference locally was to try and improve the flow of young people through our service. It seems sometimes that we're not as efficient as we could be about the work we do. We want to give the highest quality care to young people. But this has led to long waiting lists and some overwork, where we keep offering families sessions even when there's been progress, because it can be really hard to let people go. Or we struggle to discharge young people from our inpatient unit because we can't get the right people to attend the discharge meeting. As part of the GenerationQ process I had learned about Lean, and it made me think how similar it was to a process that exists in child mental health services called the Choice and Partnership Approach (CAPA). This approach combines personalised care and collaborative practice with the people using the service. It was developed by two child and adolescent psychiatrists, Ann York and Steve Kingsbury, and has been widely used in children and young people's mental health settings in the UK. It appealed to me as an approach because it supports service transformation by demanding a change in philosophy, rather than being simply a set of quality improvement tools.

Why Lean?

As I understand it, Lean as a quality improvement approach is not usually associated with mental health services, although there is growing interest in this area. I am drawn to Lean philosophies and methods in my area of work, as I appreciate the focus on looking after the workforce for sustainable organisations, and the concept of focusing on value to the user of the service is very important to me. Although some have criticised the use of the term "customer" when considering Lean thinking in health care, I like it, because I think the use of this language shifts the focus of what "value" really means to a young person or family. For too long, leaders in health services have been focused on what *they* value as the "experts", not what patients really want and need. To me, it is of critical importance that clinicians support young people to identify what value means to them when using services, and doing this by setting "Goal Based Outcomes" (Law 2015) – a way of asking young people and families what they think would be a good outcome for them. Without this information, we are at risk of disempowering an already marginalised group, and providing treatment "to" young people rather than with them. There is then huge potential for waste from young people not attending appointments, continuing to keep appointments for longer than necessary, and delayed discharges from hospital and services working to commissioning targets rather than those of the patient. I feel that there can be a clinical risk of poor outcomes from people dropping out of treatment because it is not what they wanted or needed (but they might feel unable to say), or people attending treatment but just not getting better because it is not the right treatment for them.

Leading, according to Lean philosophy, requires forming good relationships, but the concept of flow also seems relevant to my work context. Traditionally, young people's mental health services have been characterised by long waiting lists for initial assessments, then long internal waits for a specialist clinician or treatment. We know that the longer young people wait for mental health treatment the worse their symptoms become, but services are now caught in a negative cycle where they cannot offer early intervention because they are focused on all the people who have been waiting a long time to be seen. These people have often deteriorated whilst on the waiting list, and consequently require more intensive and longer treatment than they would if they had been seen sooner. For example, a young person referred by their GP for low mood and some self-harm might be supported to manage their mood and find alternative methods of emotion regulation if they are seen by a mental health professional in a timely manner. However, if they are left waiting, for up to a year in some cases, without professional support their difficulties and hopelessness can grow, often into self-medicating behaviour such as using drugs or alcohol, and more significant self-harm, as well as reduced functioning such as not attending school.

Leading for quality

My primary intention with this work was to improve the quality of the child and adolescent mental health service in terms of efficiency and outcomes. I also wanted to understand a bit more about my own leadership and how I could be more effective. I was participating on a leadership programme, GenerationQ, and so the reading and the conversations were prompting questions in my head. I found myself struggling to stop being the person who "did the doing". It felt hard to step back, to be setting the strategic direction and coaching others to implement the required changes. I found myself in a vicious cycle of taking on too much, feeling overwhelmed, then not being as effective or impactful at work or at home. I had a self-narrative of taking on responsibility for everything that happened to me and every-thing I was involved in, rather than understanding my place in a social context where I am both influencing of and influenced by others. I also had a sense of not quite knowing when and how I was most effective or powerful, therefore where to focus my energies. My hope was that by introducing a set of principles and a way of thinking about how to improve quality through improving flow, I would be able to lead a multi-disciplinary group of clinicians to create better outcomes for young people who needed our services.

When I was planning to introduce the ideas of Lean into the service, I was struck by an anxiety about how my actions would be interpreted by my colleagues. I was in no way an expert on quality improvement, and I wondered if they might think I was overstepping the line, trying to get involved in something that wasn't my role. I remembered a time earlier in my career when I had been criticised by a senior manager for being "too ambitious". Although I was an experienced doctor in a position of responsibility and power, I took this criticism to heart as a form of shame. It made me want to draw back into myself and give up attempting to improve the service. I felt I should just get on with my clinical work and stop trying to make changes. Later, I discovered Sheryl Sandberg's book *Lean In* (2015) and read about how other women have experienced similar gender stereotyping and been called "ambitious" or "pushy" when they are trying to make a difference.

Learning to embrace my passion and ambition, whilst acknowledging their shadow sides, was to be an important part of my leadership development process. So was acknowledging my vulnerability. I discovered Brené Brown's work on shame and vulnerability (Brown 2012) and it really helped me understand that one of the main consequences of feeling shame was to reduce my connection to colleagues, for fear of being vulnerable and open to further attack.

The first meeting

Reflecting on the memory of that incident earlier in my career, and discussing my feelings with my GenerationQ action learning group, I was able to acknowledge my anxieties about being an imposter in quality improvement, and decided I still wanted to put my proposal for this work to my service's clinical leadership team. One thing I had learned was not to try and go it alone! I met with Emma and Robert, the Senior Manager and Nursing Lead to propose a project. I really wanted to engage them in this work and inspire a passion in them for quality improvement, not just quality assurance. I find that I can be quite sensitive to criticism, especially from Robert. It feels sometimes that I bring too much energy to our conversations, and when he adopts a cautious position I end up deflated. One example of this was when I came back from a conference and suggested we look at the use of digital technology to interact with our patients online. Robert said that this had been tried before and it just wasn't safe. I felt slightly foolish and wondered if I'd rushed in too quickly with this idea. I knew that I needed to connect with them this time if this was going to work but I also needed to have confidence in my position to influence change.

I introduced the idea of looking more closely at how we worked together to implement Lean (in the form of the Choice and Partnership Approach) and wondered what their best hopes would be for the project. Emma said she hoped we would be able to use data in a more helpful way, and that this would allow us to communicate to commissioners and executives in the Trust about how hard we were trying to reduce waiting times. Robert said that he hoped the introduction of the processes would support staff to feel less overwhelmed with workloads, particularly the nursing staff. I agreed and added that my hope focused on value to the young person and ensuring that whatever we do is as efficient as can be. We agreed that we would devote our next meeting to liaising with the different clinical leads to engage them in thinking about Lean as a way of improving flow and increasing capacity in our service. It was essential that they were part of shaping these developments.

Reflecting on this conversation, I was clear that I was trying to improve my relationship with Robert in particular by connecting with him and his priorities. I was frustrated that he seemed focused on his staff group (nursing) when I saw that we had a responsibility for all our staff – as well as our patients! However, he appeared to be interested in the work so I was keen to build on his interest. Emma seemed quite engaged, and had mentioned to me afterwards how she thought it could make a significant difference to waiting times. I noticed how we each had different priorities for the project. Emma wanted data for commissioners, Robert wanted to ensure staff were protected from unrealistic workload expectations, and I wanted to improve flow. These differences may have gone unnoticed if I had not explicitly asked for everyone's ideas before expressing my own. This felt different to our usual interactions, and it made me think that often I am so keen to get the job done I may state my agenda first, preventing others from feeling that they can disagree.

The second meeting

My next challenge was going to be engaging the clinical leads. The purpose of the meeting with them was to reach consensus about how best to implement the improvement process. I reflected on how to approach this meeting, and noticed that I felt a strong urge to tell people what to do, to use my power as the leader to "prescribe" the solution to our improvement problem (Heron 2009). I understood this was linked to my anxiety about getting results around this project. Clinically, I know that a drive for control is a common reaction if someone is fearful of the future being negative, and that this is often stronger if that person believes the responsibility for the outcome is solely theirs. My personal script about an internal locus of control has served me well in helping me believe that I can achieve my goals, but I was beginning to see the shadow side of over-responsibility which comes to the fore when I am under pressure.

Identifying and choosing not to act on my urge to control the meeting gave me the chance to experiment with leading in a different and new way. And of course, if the staff weren't engaged with the whole purpose of what we were trying to achieve, it wouldn't be sustained anyway. I wanted them to bring their own expert knowledge of what might work in the teams, so framed the conversation as a way of thinking together. My role was to hold enough uncertainty to enable a generative conversation, to use my listening and reflecting skills, and to deliberately offer the staff group the power to decide where to start with Lean.

I wanted to set the context and find common ground between us, so I started by asking the group what they thought was the purpose of our work, what were we trying to do. One of the group responded, "We are trying to improve the mental health of children and young people. Or are we? Should we be focusing on a small group with severe needs?" This started a discussion about what work we should prioritise in the context of reducing budgets. It exposed different beliefs people had about the purpose and therefore nature of our work, which seemed to be based on their values, professional background and experience. This in turn led to a wider reflection in the group about increasing demand for child and adolescent mental health services, due to increasing rates of mental health difficulties in young people and reducing support services because of budget cuts. What emerged from this activity was an acknowledgement that, as a service, we would never be able to meet the full demand of all young people and families who wanted support – we had to agree, with commissioners and our service user group, on priorities. The group decided on the elements of Lean that they wanted to start with, and they made an action plan for these tasks. Crucially, they all agreed that it would be a helpful thing to do, and they made a commitment to embed the new processes in the teams.

Afterwards, I thought about what I had learned from this, about how I use my power as a leader. I realised that I had been anxious about stating my position explicitly for fear that it would dampen others' expressions of opinion. I also reflected, however, that advocating for something, in this case the implementation of Lean principles and processes, is not the same as imposing my will. My role meant that I had the power to call the meeting, set the agenda and expect people to attend. Taking the role of facilitator had meant that I was using relational power (and skills) to guide the conversation and regulate the emotional atmosphere in the room. I had been able to create a space of safe uncertainty, and to accept that, as a leader, I am not responsible for the whole service but I am responsible for creating the conditions in which it can thrive and productive conversations can take place.

Absence

Not long after this meeting, I became ill. Lying in my hospital bed I began to wonder how I had got there. Firstly, I was noticing the narrative around my illness. Most people I spoke to said, "Oh have you been doing too much again?" which I found quite critical, and I didn't like the implication that the illness was my fault. However, on further reflection I was able to accept that I had been working very hard and this had probably been a contributing factor.

Just before I became ill, I had received some feedback as part of my appraisal. It had been an interesting session as the feedback from my colleagues had been so overwhelmingly positive, not only about my skills and abilities but also my personal qualities such as kindness and care. These qualities were values of mine, but had become subordinate narratives in my sense of self as a leader. The feedback enabled me to remember that these qualities are part of my authentic self, and who I am is actually my greatest asset as a leader! There were several comments in the feedback that referred to me "doing too much" and "needing to achieve a work life balance". Looking back on these comments made me realise that over-estimating my personal capacity had been a blind spot for me, but was known to others. I was later able to reflect that my drive to achieve and get things done can result in burnout, but can also look to others like I am unable to make priorities and set boundaries on this basis. Not only does this reduce my presence, it also reduces my potency.

When I began my phased return to work, I noticed something different in my colleagues and in me. I had been ill, I still felt vulnerable, and I was received back in the service literally with open arms. It was clear that people had keenly felt my absence which was surprising and humbling. I realised that I wasn't just a cog in a wheel, a set of technical skills; I meant something to the people I worked with, whether as a leader, a team member or a human being.

Outcome

In order to evaluate progress with this project, the teams completed a self-assessment rating scale about which elements of Lean they had adopted. We found that before the improvement project, teams were only using 6/20 (30 percent) of the elements of Lean we had agreed to use, but by the time of my return teams were using 17/20 (85 percent) of the elements. This has since led to a significant reduction in waiting times for the service and a shift in culture, with clinicians talking about, and paying attention to, ideas of flow and quality improvement.

Reflection

My experience of leading a quality improvement project in a children and young people's mental health service taught me that developing relationships with all the staff involved was central to the process. I started off afraid of my positional and expert power as personal dominant narratives, but I seemed to have forgotten about the warm, trusting relationships I am able to form with colleagues. My appraisal process reminded me of this; it was also reinforced through conversations with Emma about how our good working relationship enabled us to share power in jointly leading the service. I believe that Emma and I have a particular commitment to this relationship; connecting with her has been a big part of this learning for me, and I am building on this experience to connect more with Robert.

I have experimented with improving connection with all of my colleagues and being my authentic warm self. It has been a joy to develop my working relationships further. I discovered that deliberately taking a facilitative style with colleagues was a powerful leadership gesture. I learned that my Hurry Up driver [see Appendix 3] and sense of responsibility was often driving my tendency to take on too much and do things myself. By consciously slowing down I was able to share decision-making power with colleagues, who then themselves took the responsibility for outcomes. This felt like me taking what Transactional Analysis (Lapworth and Sills 2011) would consider an Adult/Adult approach rather than a Parent/Child dynamic [see Appendix 2]. The drive to take a directive, parental role in the past may have been driven by anxiety, but also by a need to prove my authority.

Throughout this process I have learnt about complexity thinking and the importance of paying attention to our gestures and how others respond. By paying attention to this level of interpersonal interaction I have found a shift in my relationships which has led to a richer quality of dialogue and quite rapid changes. The value of being present emerged during this project, and a discovery that my presence as a leader was important to my colleagues. I have learned that my skills lie not only in my technical ability, but also in my relational skills and growing understanding of myself. The theme of priorities and how to make choices emerged throughout this project. It seems to me that these complex issues deserve a dialogue approach, where leaders can sit with the uncertainty, resist the pull for control and order, and engage staff and service users in thinking about these dilemmas. I also need to consider what my priorities are for my own limited capacity.

I called this chapter *Leaning Out and Letting Go* because for women leaders in the NHS it is not as simple as "leaning in". In my experience, and listening to other female colleagues, we are often criticised for being ambitious or pushy, labels rarely applied to male colleagues in a negative way. One response to this criticism is to disconnect from our colleagues and "get the job done". But this isn't right either. We can't detach ourselves from our colleagues, however painful the experience is sometimes. The only way to achieve our aims is to work them out together. Most people who choose to work in the National Health Service do so from a desire to help others and improve lives. Those who choose to lead in the NHS also often have this drive, but it can be a difficult position to take. By bringing our "selves" to work, remaining authentic and connected to colleagues as well as service users, we are more able to make informed decisions to maximise the quality of care we give to ourselves as well as others.

I'd like to finish this chapter with an extract from writing by Marianne Williamson (1992), which has also been used by Nelson Mandela to express some of our dilemmas when thinking about our own power.

> *Our deepest fear is not that we are inadequate. Our deepest fear is that we are powerful beyond measure. It is our light, not our darkness that most frightens us. We ask ourselves, 'Who am I to be brilliant, gorgeous, talented, fabulous?' Actually, who are you not to be? … as we let our own light shine, we unconsciously give other people permission to do the same. As we are liberated from our own fear, our presence automatically liberates others.*

Marianne Williamson 1992, p. 190

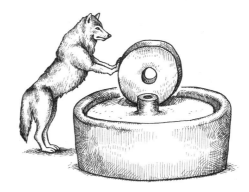

CHAPTER 11

Joining the Pack

A wake-up call

Imagine the scene. I am sitting across the table from the Director of Strategy of a major charity. Sitting alongside her are three of her colleagues. The pot of coffee is on the table, ready to pour. They are here at my invitation to talk about my idea of setting up a regional Quality Improvement (QI) Academy for my specialty. I hope that they will support the project. I don't know the Director, who is new in post, or her colleagues, but I have heard that she is keen to bring the ideas of quality improvement into her organisation. We shake hands, pour the coffee and all sit somewhat awkwardly on the edge of our seats. Who is going to speak first?

I jump in. I haven't prepared a presentation or an agenda, but I am keen to share my thinking. As I start I am aware I am speaking quickly, perhaps too quickly, and yet I am so full of excitement, so convinced about the merits of my idea, that I press on.

"This is the opportunity to create something really exciting, something new, and a major change for our specialism. Too often we focus on introducing new services and yet there is so much untapped opportunity to improve what we already do. I have a vision for what it could be like. We could trial a range of improvement methods. I am sure that you will agree with me that..."

I noticed that the Director was looking down at her notebook. I felt a pang of concern that she might not be listening to me.

"That's interesting. I was wondering whether you might be able to help me prepare some documents for our charity's new strategy. Your input would be welcome."

Now I was the one at risk of not listening.

"Yes. Yes of course. Although the idea of being experimental and trialling an Academy..."

One of the Director's colleagues spoke up:

"Why don't you send us a proposal, in writing?"

I did. I didn't receive a response.

I felt mortified. Why hadn't they bought my great idea? I knew that they had available funds. I am sure my enthusiasm and commitment shone through. It was a great idea – the opportunity to transform how we support people at the end of their life. What could be more important?

I felt the shame begin to creep up on me, a pattern I recognise in myself when I feel I have done something wrong, or worse still, failed. Had I not presented my case compellingly enough? Was my vision not grand enough? Should I have been more forceful and sold my ideas more convincingly?

As painful as it was at the time, reflecting upon this event with the challenge and support of my action learning set colleagues (I was participating in the GenerationQ programme at the time) was the beginning of a personal wake-up call, and a shift in how I see myself as a leader. Looking back now, the seeds of my failure to gain support in this instance are evident: it was all about me. My vision, my project, my need to be listened to and hammer home my ideas and, accompanying this, my responsibility to make it happen. And maybe too, I was neither as certain nor confident as I had tried to portray.

The time had come to understand more about this encounter and more about myself if I was going to be successful in setting up a Quality Academy.

In this chapter, my intention is to share my story of learning how not to be a lone wolf, of learning how to reach out and involve others in the practice of improvement; learning how to join the pack rather than staying separate from it. Sometimes when we look back on events and talk about them to others, it's tempting to tell the story as if the events unfolded in a smooth, planned way, with very few difficulties along the way. Having such a retrospective view enables us to show (or pretend!) that we were really in control all along, and that we set the goal and achieved it.

In truth, we all know that life and work is seldom like this. When I look back over my attempts to set up a Quality Academy – which I have done, by the way – I realise that there was no smooth path, but rather one with plenty of bumps, and I nearly fell over some of them while some gave me an unexpected lift. I think that the best way to tell my story is to explore some of those bumps, and how they affected me and the progress of this project, to share some of my "moments of truth" and the learning that flowed from them.

Listening and inquiry matters

If the encounter with the national charity was the first moment of truth, I learned a great deal. On GenerationQ I had read a lot about the art of dialogue and the importance of really listening and inquiring into others' points of view. In this encounter I experienced the impact of not doing either. Looking back now, I had entered the room with frozen thoughts. There was not room in either my mind or the conversation for me to adjust my position, change my perspective or learn from the other. I had been so caught up in advocating my position and hammering home my agenda that I had not stopped and truly listened, nor inquired into how the other attendees were seeing the world. As a result, I had not developed any kind of relationship with these people – why should they trust me and my ideas?

Facing personal daemons

I also learned a lot about my own personal drivers and motivations and how they can trip me up, as well as serve me well. The theoretical concept of personal drivers is explained in Appendix 3 although I personally find it helpful to liken them to Philip Pullman's idea of daemons as he writes about in his Dark Materials Trilogy. Put simply, the concept is that in adult life some of our behaviour stems from behavioural patterns which were established and appropriate in childhood as we learned how to behave in order to be accepted by those around us. Typically, these patterns continue to serve us well in adulthood but, if overdone, can become a rod for our own backs.

For me, I realised that two of the five drivers have a tendency to dominate my behaviour and they both played out in the encounter: Try Hard, and Hurry Up. The first, Try Hard, was established in childhood and reinforced throughout study, qualification and then clinical practice. The underpinning belief is that I will always do well, if only I *try harder*, that "more" is always needed if I am to be "good enough". In certain circumstances, this belief has really served me well. It has motivated me to put in the hours, to push on in the service of patients. The shadow side, however, is that in this encounter I was – perhaps unconsciously – on the lookout for a trophy project, a big one, where I could get the accolade and the affirmation that I was indeed trying hard enough. Combined with my Hurry Up driver I felt compelled to act big and act fast – no time to waste on building relationships, taking people with me or starting small. I have since learned to notice when I am in the grip of these drivers, to give myself choice in how I respond.

I also reflected that my own uncertainty and nervousness about setting up an Academy had led me to seek external recognition, rather than trust myself. If I could set up a big project with the support of a large national charity, it would go some way to proving this was the right thing to be doing. In this encounter, I had not been brave enough to let them see my vulnerability, that I needed their collaboration, maybe their help. I had hidden behind a false bravado. I will go on to say more about this, about how choosing to sometimes let your vulnerability be seen can be the right thing to do.

Gaining senior level support

The outcome of the meeting with the national charity had rather knocked my confidence, but I was determined to keep going, to find a way to bring an improvement focus into the organisation. Up to this point, I had seen the establishment of an academy as a pretty single-handed venture. Of course, others might be interested, but I was carrying the responsibility for making it happen – alone. Looking back now I can see that I was still very attached to a heroic model of leadership.

However, my thinking was beginning to shift. Reflecting upon the meeting and my participation on GenerationQ was beginning to make me question this heroic vision of leadership. I began to realise that although, in my experience, this style of leadership is widespread in health care, it has not always been the most successful. In addition, when overdone it has led to burnout for leaders, and a sense of disempowerment or coercion of those being led.

I decided that I would try a different approach. Together, my growing evangelism for QI and my Hurry Up driver were creating growing pressure inside me to do something. I organised a QI introductory lecture and invited all the organisation's trustees, the executive team and the directors from our Health and Social Care partners. As I write this, I can't help but smile and reflect that patterns are hard to shift. Despite lessons from the first moment of truth, here I was once again "going big", hoping to secure that trophy project by reaching out and inviting all the big guns to my first venture. It could have gone horribly wrong.

Thankfully, it didn't. Despite my ambition I was feeling far from confident to deliver the lecture myself, and so invited a colleague from GenerationQ with years of QI experience to do it for me. She was fabulous, holding her expertise lightly and engaging the audience in discussion. I could feel their growing excitement about the potential to improve patient care and I received good feedback about the event afterwards. This was salutary and positive learning for me that leadership isn't always about being at the front, but sometimes involves creating space for others to shine. I decided to invite the CEO and Vice Chairman of the Board to join me in gathering ideas by visiting an organisation similar to our own which had embraced QI.

Seeing QI in practice was helpful, but it was not the big win of the trip. More important was the conversation we had on the train coming home together. As the CEO said as we went our separate ways home at the station:

"I love it. Having now seen what is possible, we must do it...let's press ahead."

This conversation was my second "moment of truth" and this time it felt good. Not only did I now have the ear and support of the senior team, I was beginning to feel no longer alone. The "I" had become "we" and I had recruited my first followers. I had begun the transformation from an individual with an idea, into a leader, albeit a tentative one.

Building momentum

I now began to think more carefully about the form and approach this Quality Academy might take. I was not attracted to the idea of offering somewhat dry sessions on theory with little or no practical application. Instead, I was moving towards wanting to find a way to combine structured instruction about the various improvement methods with experiential learning. Ultimately, I hoped to establish an academy capable of developing skilled improvement coaches who would then subsequently recruit followers themselves. I was still feeling that my own QI knowledge was not sufficient to undertake the training and development needed, so I began searching for "QI experts" who could deliver the initial workshops for me. When I reflect on this time, I notice an interesting apparent contradiction in my thinking. On the one hand, I wanted to launch something big, to be seen as the one heading up a trophy project. I wanted to show others (and perhaps myself) that I was capable and knowledgeable about Quality Improvement.

On the other hand, in secret, I felt distinctly lacking in expertise and therefore in confidence. What did I know compared to those people I had met who had years of quality improvement experience under their belts? If I tried to lead an academy myself, my lack of knowledge would surely be exposed.

Following encouragement from colleagues on the GenerationQ programme, I saw that my search for the expert was most probably a deep-rooted fear of failure and a lack of understanding about my own sources of power and credibility. The risk of shame and my inner voice telling me that I wasn't good enough to have a go at teaching, even though my colleagues reassured me that I was completely capable, were paralysing me. I chose to take my first true step into the unknown, to trust that I had acquired sufficient knowledge and skills to lead a QI training programme, and to let myself learn from the experience; to risk getting it wrong.

With much trepidation, I put three dates for a "Quality Improvement Group" (QIG) in the diary and invited any interested staff to join in. To my delight, 13 colleagues accepted; nurses, managers, a doctor, social workers, administrators, and even the CEO!

At this stage I was still not sure what we might cover or how. I was surprised to notice that my fear was beginning to turn to excitement and that I had a growing sense of trust in what was rapidly becoming an emergent process.

On the day of the first QIG I arrived at work without knowing how I had got there. With hindsight, I probably wasn't a very safe cyclist that morning – my mind was elsewhere. How had I, a clinician, got to this point? What on earth was I up to? Those voices of self-doubt were loud in my head. The room looked great. It was full of light, just a simple circle of chairs and a couple of flip-charts. Everyone turned up. Unlike that first meeting with the charity, this time I was determined to start well by giving time to the group to establish itself, for us to find out a bit more about each other and why we had each chosen to show up. In my back pocket I had lots of ideas about how to teach the group about the IHI Model of Improvement and the concept of PDSA cycles, but I was determined to keep that Hurry Up driver at bay.

To my joy, the first session worked well, and people commented that they had enjoyed the open interaction and the sense that I had not been holding pre-determined ideas about what the outcome of the meeting would be. I enjoyed it too, appreciating the growing energy in the room, the sense of shared excitement. I got to teach the QI models and we had a good discussion about how we might each – and together – put them to the test in our own organisation. I have read recently that leadership is sometimes about *convening*. I had just convened our first QI meeting and, pushing back against that disabling inner voice, I was also beginning to believe that I might be good enough, expert enough, to do it and take it forward.

Taking a personal risk

So, we had begun, and things were going well. After two sessions we had understood about the concept of quality, and people had been introduced to the Model for Improvement. A few had even told stories of their experiments and challenges with PDSA cycles. Yet somehow, I still felt distant from those I desperately wanted to join with me, and lacking in confidence that they would stay the course, that the improvement efforts would be sustained. I was struggling with how to really engage and feel connected, and how to build a sense of trust among us.

A key shift occurred when I learnt about how vulnerability can become the "birthplace of innovation, creativity and change" (Brown 2010) and how both vulnerability and humility can be valuable to create connection. With a metaphorical intake of breath, I realised that I needed the QIG group more than they needed me. Reframing it in this way helped me prepare for future encounters with more humility.

At the start of one meeting, once we had got to know each other a little more, I chose to reveal that I had even considered cancelling the meeting, so strong was my sense of uncertainty, nervousness and fear of failure. I must have been true in my gesture (in my word and intention) as it evoked a sincere and Adult (in Transactional Analysis terms) response, without a hint of them needing to rescue me.

"Because you say it with sincerity. What I hear you say and see you do are congruent .... It makes it feel genuine."

"The way you were so open, in asking for our help, made us want to help."

"You are very human. You just bring out the best in us. Because we aren't afraid to try."

Another moment of truth. By now I had completely abandoned any notion that I was on top or in control. This removed a huge burden of responsibility from my shoulders. I no longer needed to predict the future, achieve perfection and know the answers. I found this very liberating. As Goffee (2005, p. 64) wrote, "If they think you are perfect they will leave you to do it!" I hope and believe my new found way of being and my actions also relieved others of their need to be perfect. My willingness to learn created space for mutual learning. I was feeling both more real and more human, and the need for any trophy project or external affirmation was beginning to slip away. As one of the complexity thinkers writes, "The more we realise that we do not know exactly what to do, the greater the risk and anticipation and the more stimulated we become". (Shaw 2002, p. 14)

Creating a shared vision

After six QIG meetings I invited the group to review the programme and join me in developing our Quality Vision for the organisation. I offered a first draft. As people started suggesting changes to my first draft – just what I had asked them to do – I was taken aback by my reaction. I felt resistant, almost indignant that they might disagree with how I had seen the future. Patterns are indeed hard to shift, and it seemed I still had some letting go to do!

By now though, the group had life and spirit of its own and we had become peers. I had invited difference and diversity of view and experience and now I needed to respect it. I felt truly elated as a shared vision and unshakeable commitment emerged from conversations during two further meetings. We had lost some people on the way. Of the original 13 recruits, not all finished the course. But enough did and wanted to play a role in supporting the vision they had co-created. They were no longer first followers but new leaders, and some went on to use their experiences to co-design the next iteration of the programme.

I had started out with the perspective of what I would do to others: I would teach them, and they would learn. Yet the process became as much about my learning as it was that of others. This occurred through learning to listen to and value other perspectives, channelling the richness of the diversity and reflecting together on the way. We ended up as co-educators. Whilst I might have set a direction, bringing people along was achieved through creating a space to come together, building relationships and encouraging conversations.

I haven't disguised just how anxious I felt at times. Was all the time and effort worthwhile? When I was least expecting it (and perhaps no longer needing it quite as much) the external affirmation I had started off by craving, came my way. The CEO described the QI programme as "An excellent achievement," and reassured me that "A large effort is initially needed to get a millstone turning, but once rotating it requires much less to maintain." I rather like that metaphor.

Coming close to derailment

My keenness to lead with and through others nearly became derailed when the trustees, enthused by what they were hearing, requested a formal QI strategy. As to be expected by now, I responded with my Hurry Up and Try Hard drivers, fuelled further by yet another driver – Please Others – which is often hooked by requests from others. Within days I had sourced and was modifying a written QI strategy from a high-achieving NHS Trust. I also began to think about proposing a budget for a new QI expert. I was in the grip of a familiar pattern to act alone, at speed, and to believe that expertise was what was needed here.

Only through challenge (again) from my GenerationQ colleagues did I recognise, and then challenge, my own assumption that good QI leaders must personally write the QI strategy. I was failing to apply, or turn to, any of the theories which I had been learning. I rushed headlong into action, following my natural tendency to think alone and to have all the answers. Fortunately my GenerationQ colleagues had "caught me" just in time. If I had pressed on I was at risk of embarking on a trajectory where I was trying to predict the unpredictable and, in the process, leave everyone else behind. My strategy would likely fail, or simply be superseded by events. But how could I report to the trustees that I would not write a QI strategy?

I began to think that there might be a middle way. To satisfy the need for something deliberate, to contain all our anxiety, but without committing to a predetermined future, I wrote something which complexity thinkers refer to as a "minimum specification" (McCandless 2008). This described the process for creating the conditions for continuous quality improvement. I argued that the QI strategy outcome would unfold in time. My role would be as an enabler. This approach would be risky – what response might it evoke? – but I was ready to give it a try.

The pressure was again lifted from my shoulders. I reached out to the QIG group and shared the responsibility to co-create this specification, and to my delight no one seemed to think any less of my abilities. It meant embracing a significant degree of uncertainty, but it was worth it as by now I was convinced it was more likely to result in a useful and sustainable strategy.

My need for a trophy project had gone and the trustees embraced the document.

Unintended consequences

All was beginning to go well. I had relieved myself of the need to be a heroic, all-knowing leader, and had found unexpected and delightful support from those I was working with. But my peace was to be short-lived.

Stephen burst into my office.

"Thank you for making me appear useless at my job!"

Despite all my rhetoric about expecting the unexpected, I hadn't bargained for this. Stephen had been a fellow director for several years. I knew that he was struggling to understand my new role as the quality improvement lead, but I was shocked by these words and perhaps even more by the tears which followed. Once the initial surprise had passed, I began to inquire into the reasons for his anger and upset.

"The creation of a Quality Academy is a sure signal to the organisation that my area has poor quality and that you have been forced to step in. To take over."

Of course, we spent some time examining this and both apologising to and reassuring each other. We both valued our relationship too much to let this upset be ignored or brushed to one side.

I tell this story because of its impact on me. It helped me recognise the unintended consequences of my actions. Although my intention was to help others strive for excellence, I was aware that I had a tendency at times to stray into being unappreciative of others, or unintentionally self-promoting. As a result, I can undermine others' self-value. In doing so my actions weaken my intentions of improving patient care, replacing this with an unhelpful and unconscious desire for affirmation. Unwittingly this can make some people less inclined to receive the intended help. This was the antithesis of what I was seeking to achieve, and it seemed as if this was just what had happened between Stephen and me.

Once again, in an uncomfortably real way, I could see the impact on others of me not feeling good enough about myself. This can lead me all too easily to compete with others in order to try to see myself in a better light, to miss the value and richness of others' views, to take up the role of Critical Parent or rescuer in the drama triangle [see Appendix 2], and, worst of all, to perceive colleagues who become too skilled as threats.

My moment of truth with Stephen led to some deep soul searching. It led me to question whether I wanted to lead improvement to make me feel good, or because I wanted the organisation to succeed and the quality of care to get even better.

I began to challenge myself. Could I shift, or quieten, my need for external recognition? Understanding the part recognition plays in my life, and working with it, offered me a chance at a greater autonomy than I had ever experienced. My happiness and success were in my own hands.

I started by working hard at crediting, celebrating and joining in others' successes – not always successfully, but I think I am improving. I have also become more aware of the social level messages and their ability to help and hinder. The Please Others driver can be helpful in establishing clinical relationships with patients and staff, but can encourage heroic or rescuing leadership. The Hurry Up driver promotes speedy results and a willingness to experiment rather than wait for perfection, but also puts pressure on others and can result in leading alone. I can't change my natural instincts, but I can learn to notice them and use them choicefully. I can turn a "demon" with a negative connotation into a daemon, or virtue, which I can appreciate.

The last time I spoke with Stephen, I shared with him that I was new to this QI leadership role and that his honesty had really helped me realise that I didn't always get it right, and how I may at times make people feel. I explained to him what I thought I would like to offer in the post, explained how I hoped I could do this, and asked him whether he would be prepared to support me and work with me. He said he would, and I then asked him if he would be willing to continue giving me frank feedback. I noticed that he seemed to feel good about the conversation and the request, and this made me feel good too!

A parallel transition

At the start of this project I thought I would be taking others through a transition, where they would come to see QI as part of their work. Now, I see my own transition running in parallel. I am transitioning from being primarily a clinical practitioner to a new beginning as a leader of QI. The emerging success of the QI programme prompted the trustees and CEO to encourage me to drop most clinical roles and adopt, almost full time, a facilitative leadership role to shift the culture of the organisation to be more conducive to and capable of improvement.

Through the QI work, I have glimpsed a new horizon filled with opportunities, fulfilment, and the chance of personal growth, yet with an area of vulnerability. My identity is shifting and that is both challenging and frightening. However, I have chosen to take the risk, as the opportunity to grow from where I am now to somewhere new, and the possibility of innovation, excite me.

Credit belongs to the man ...., if he fails, at least fails while daring greatly, so that his place shall never be with those cold and timid souls who neither know victory nor defeat.

Roosevelt (1910)

I am proud to say that there are growing signs all around me of a commitment to make QI more centre stage. I have been supported to appoint a locum consultant to take on much of my clinical role to free up my time to lead on QI, and I am working with fellow directors and the CEO to develop realistic shared objectives for how we can use these new approaches. Our trustees too want to lend their support to the "massive changes" in culture that they are already experiencing.

Whilst this is a great start, much remains to do and learn, and there is much uncertainty about the best ways to get there. Yet, since the best parts of my learning have been those aspects I could not have imagined or planned beforehand, this seems an exciting prospect. I expect that I will make mistakes, but somehow this feels exciting too since with each lies the opportunity to learn and become better. Perhaps at some point I will no longer need to seek affirmation – it will find me.

Committing
Working at scale

The first set of stories described the early, often tentative, steps in an improvement project, as a phase of experimenting. The next set of stories gives accounts of trying to get something going on a larger scale. This last selection of stories is from Fellows who have found themselves in a context, and at a time, where something larger still is possible.

To create the conditions in which a philosophy of improvement and patient experience can flourish organisation wise is hard work and requires tenacity and resilience, as well as board level support and commitment.

There are three stories in this section:
- The first, *Improvement Is the Work*, details the decision and the steps involved when a Trust decides to wholeheartedly embrace a quality improvement methodology, in this case Lean. There are difficulties and resistance along the way, and it takes a whole new way of working for everyone to really embrace this approach.
- The second, *Daisy*, is a story about the way a bottom-up safety initiative spread throughout a hospital.
- The third, *A Thread of Kindness*, concerns the refocusing of an organisation towards a much more patient-driven perspective of health care. Even with an extraordinary level of support from the board, the Fellow begins modestly, knowing that to overreach could stop this improvement in its tracks. As things begin to gather momentum, there is still the need to have some honest

conversations about areas of the Trust where compassionate care seemed to be lacking

These stories provides a link or segue from this book, *Beyond the Toolkit*, to its companion, *Hope Behind the Headlines*. The theme of how improving quality requires "shifting the culture", altering the dominant way in which people behave and think, is explained in further detail in *Hope Behind the Headlines*, along with reflections about some of the challenges and successes in making this shift.

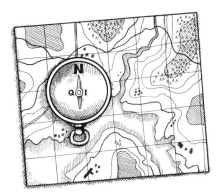

CHAPTER 12

Improvement Is the Work

I knew that I wanted to move to a new organisation. I was restless and, when honest with myself, frustrated where I was. I could see so many opportunities to improve the quality of care we offered our patients and I did what I could to make a difference, pushing here, nudging there, offering my support to others who I noticed also trying to lead improvement. And yet, it felt piecemeal, as if we were paying lip service to making quality of care central to all our activities. As hard as I tried, and I did try hard, to influence the senior execs to make quality improvement (QI) centre stage, I failed. Looking back now, with the benefit of hindsight, I think I can understand why, and it's a bigger issue than just the organisation I was in at the time, or my influencing tactics – more on that later.

I began to cautiously look around for a new job. I knew by this time that the context and culture of an organisation matter; they can make the difference between improvement efforts becoming mainstream or efforts stalling. I had two criteria in mind as I searched. Firstly, I was looking for a Trust that was stable enough and not in the depths of financial crisis, as otherwise it would be too difficult to make the sort of changes that I wanted to see. I was also searching for kindred spirits, a leadership team that shared my values and aspiration for making quality improvement the focus for leading the organisation. When I showed up to interviews it had to be a two-way street: was I right for this organisation and was this organisation right for me? After several false starts I found myself sitting in front of an interview panel and the question they were keen to explore with me was:

> So how can we develop the culture of our organisation so that quality improvement is central to everything we do?

At last! Part of me couldn't believe that this was finally happening. The panel seemed genuinely interested in an exploratory conversation, not constrained by the more typical competency-based interviews I had experienced elsewhere. I knew there and then that this was the place I wanted to be, the work I wanted to commit to, and I felt a real thrill of excitement, a sense of beginning to come alive again.

That was three years ago; the time has flown by and the work has been, and continues to be, a joy, although not without its ups and downs as you will hear in the story. I am a medical director, with a bit of a passion, some might call it obsession, for quality improvement. Our Trust is a medium sized acute, offering a full range of services on multiple sites. Not unlike many other acute Trusts, it is the result of a merger of two quite different and historically independent organisations. I am quite a shy and private individual and don't like talking about myself much. In fact, I am already beginning to feel rather uncomfortable as I write this. And yet, there is a story to tell here about the power of teamwork from the bottom to the top of an organisation and what can be achieved when QI *is* centre stage; when improving the quality of care *is* the work.

The story began before I arrived with the truly skilful leadership of our CEO and her team. Over a period of five or so years they had managed to turn around a pretty acrimonious merger with plenty of financial and quality problems, as well as the challenge of bringing together two different cultures. By the time I arrived they had got the house in order, achieved financial stability and Foundation Trust status. Helen, the CEO (let me call her that although it is a pseudonym), seemed to instinctively know that they had achieved base camp, but needed to up the organisation's game if they were to continue to improve. Again, instinctively, she seemed to know that quality and quality improvement were the way forward, without quite knowing what this meant in practice.

The state and status of the Trust when I arrived were great and, when I look around now, a rare gift. I was lucky indeed. We were tucked away, out of sight of London, not really on anyone's radar and we weren't raising any big red flags. Nobody was coming to interfere, and we had a sense of time and space to do what we wanted to do. The need for time and space (and trust) has become one of my mantras. When we are visited now by the great and the good, all curious to know how we have achieved what we have, looking for that silver bullet (which doesn't exist by the way), I find myself saying over and over, "Give people time and space to do what needs to be done". We don't, in my view, appoint poor leadership teams, we just don't let them do the job they need to do in the way they need to do it.

Helen was drawn to the story and work of Virginia Mason. She had met Gary Kaplan and knew something of how he had introduced Lean into what was a failing hospital in the USA. This was thinking I was very familiar with from work I had done in the past, as well as from GenerationQ. We wanted to learn more, so we had a conversation within the board and agreed to visit the Virginia Mason Institute in Seattle for a week, taking along Sarah, our OD Director who is a member of the exec team and is fabulous, and one of our senior clinicians. Even of itself, this was quite a big decision, to invest NHS cash in our own learning as well as to spend a week away from the frontline.

We learned so much from the visit and from having the opportunity to spend a week together. Yet, it wasn't so much about what they told us (you can read their journey of improvement which is available at https://www. virginiamasoninstitute.org), it was from the experience of speaking with staff, seeing and feeling the culture, touching the organisation. Everything we experienced, actions and words, breathed improvement and there was such a sense of shared ownership to do the right thing for the patient, 100 percent of the time. At the time in our hospitals I quite often witnessed patients being "passed along", becoming somebody else's problem. Here, if a problem was identified, the person who identified it held on to it and had the structures and support to improve it. The narrative was different too. I remember one fabulous conversation with a nurse in the Emergency Department. He was young, bright-eyed and hardly able to contain himself as we spoke. His excitement and enthusiasm bubbled over:

"It is just unacceptable for patients to wait, you know, unacceptable for them to wait for anything and just as unacceptable to admit a patient into the hospital without having done all our work as that would mean someone in the ward having to do our work for us."

Another big thing I noticed was that for staff at Virginia Mason, improvement was part of their core work, and they had real time to do it. So often in our NHS we start improvement projects with enthusiasm and energy but then get ground down by the sheer volume of the day-to-day.

We returned from this trip enthused, knowing that this was the kind of working practice and culture we wanted to develop, but with no idea how on earth to do it. We looked around at home but found nothing that seemed to really emulate this in the UK. It still seemed to us that most NHS organisations, even those with fabulous improvement efforts, continued to operate as if management systems and processes were separate from improvement functions and efforts. We wanted to bring the two together, but how? We knew it wasn't as simple as taking the Virginia Mason approach and implanting it in our Trust. A sure way to invite tissue rejection! We had to learn from their good practice, take faith and courage that it (something) can work and find our own way; a way that would sit well with and develop our culture at the same time.

We started with our colleagues on the board. If this was to be the long-game of improvement and culture change, we needed everyone signed up. We knew that we couldn't explain what we had experienced, that trying to sell it to the board would likely backfire and that they had to "go see it and feel it" for themselves. The Chairman and the non-execs therefore went along to visit Virginia Mason too, and what followed were three months of discussion and reflection within the board and the exec team.

This period was intense, and we had to really look at ourselves in the mirror and ask ourselves were we up to it? This was going to take significant investment in people and, perhaps most challenging of all, was going to require us to change. Many of us are traditional NHS born and bred leaders, loving nothing more than a crisis, putting on our red capes and parachuting in to fix things. This was going to require us to be different, stepping back, more facilitative, more coaching in style and tolerant of people making mistakes. Could we do it?

As a team, we decided that if we were going to do this we wanted to do it properly, not in some half-baked way, and we knew that we could not design a programme of change on our own. We needed help. We sought a partner to help us develop a bespoke Lean management system of our own, build a quality improvement function and develop internal QI capability and capacity. We recognised that we were embarking upon a three to five year programme, but were clear that we wanted to be running this ourselves within 18 months. Dependency upon external consultants, even if partners in the endeavour, was not what we wanted. In the end we chose to work with two organisations, drawn to work with the second because they got the cultural piece, the need to develop and coach people. As much as we were impressed with Virginia Mason we were wary about the dominant leadership style we had witnessed of "my way or the highway... you are either on the bus or not". We wanted something a bit softer, more people-orientated, more involving and inclusive.

Working hand in hand with our partners – by this time I and the other execs were spending at least one to two days a week on this programme – we got to work. The biggest challenge was cutting people slack and giving them time, space and support to believe it might be possible to work in this way. I can remember the first wave of ward teams we worked with. They pushed back hard:

"We don't have time for this; we absolutely don't have time given all the other stuff we have to do."

I felt some empathy, or maybe it was sympathy, at the time and fell right into the trap of trying to sell it to them. In the heat of the moment I forgot that we had spent more than three months thinking and talking. This was only the first real opportunity for the ward teams to get their heads around the ideas and think about what it would mean for them in practice. They made some compliant nods of acknowledgement, but I knew there and then that they hadn't really bought it. We had a long way to go.

We wondered and worried about what to do, knowing that any form of telling or coercion was a complete non-starter. People had to decide and choose for themselves to participate in this endeavour. We hit on the idea of asking someone else to share their experience, for us to stand back from telling. We invited a physiotherapist from one of our partner organisations, someone who had been through this first hand, to speak at our staff conference. She didn't use PowerPoint, she simply and powerfully shared her story. I think she acknowledged and legitimised how many people were feeling too. I can remember the silence in the room as she stood up to speak and a sense of anticipation. I can also remember that my heart was in my mouth. Would she be heard?

"I know that you don't believe them when they say this, but let me tell you my story, about how my day was and how frazzled I was and how I just couldn't see a way of being different. And let me describe my day now..."

I noticed that at the coffee break she was the one person that people were flocking to, curious to ask more. I need not have worried. Hearing her story was a turning point and people seemed to be beginning to believe, just a little, that change might be possible, and for the better. We then had the challenge of managing expectations amongst the exec team and the directorate divisional management teams that some things might not get done to the pace that they were used to, and that some things might not get done at all. If you invite people to take charge of what they think is important at a local level for patient care, then you must be prepared to trust them and in part let go of your own needs and agenda. One of many lessons we learned along the way.

Another turning point was when I worked with teams of nurses and doctors to focus on reducing harm, one of our key objectives. It's a long story, but it ended up with us working with ten wards with the most falls. Initially the teams responded with the usual, somewhat stuck, responses:

"*If only* we had..."

"*If only* they did ..."

Things began to shift as they worked together through their own granular data and spotted patterns, such as the importance of time of day on the frequency of falls. I can remember in one working session a real switch moment and a buzz of excitement. The energy in the room seemed to be sky-rocketing:

"You want us to design the solution?"

"You really want us to tell you how to fix it rather than be told how to fix it?"

In the space of just weeks we went from a dominant assumption of "We're a hospital full of very old people who always fall over. There's an inevitability about it", to "There's a possibility it could be different". The mood was beginning to shift as well: *this QI stuff might work.* Looking back now on this time, I can see that making sure there was no blame or, even worse, shame was so important. As was letting go of any pre-determined outcome, particularly that I might have had in mind. As a clinician pretty much addicted to fixing problems, this was personally hard going for me at times. I found myself having to literally sit on my hands.

By now, we were also starting to work hard in the exec team on our own leadership behaviours. We worked, and still do, with a team coach who joins us in action, "holds our feet to the fire", and offers us feedback, support and encouragement. We each have individual coaching sessions too. I mentioned team work at the outset of this story, and the quality of the teamwork in the exec board is one of the things that makes the work so enjoyable, as well as vital when the going gets tough. Helen has played a key role in setting the tone. When I first joined the board, I thought it a bit odd that every Tuesday morning, before the more formal meeting, we would gather together for coffee and bacon butties at 8.30am. Nobody had to tell me to come, I somehow picked up the signals that this ritual was just something we all did. Show up! I also soon learned that we didn't talk about work, we spent half an hour talking about holidays, shows, children... I joined in and yet at the back of my mind was "I've got quite a lot to do – really, do move this on". Now, in retrospect, I think that spending half an hour, once a week, just being curious about each other's lives, asking "How are you, what's going on?" has built a different kind of relationship and strong personal connections. We are colleagues and we also know each other as people. Difficult conversations are less difficult if you know the other person. From being sceptical, I now think that Helen has been really smart and that the strong personal connections we have are really, really important and core to good teamwork.

Returning to "the work", we have put into action five different "foundations", each and every one of which we now believe is important if improving the quality of patient care is to be the sustained work and focus of the organisation.

One of the foundations is Capability Development, a commitment to train and develop staff in the skills of improvement based on Lean principles. Everyone who joins the organisation has a taster session as part of their induction, and within the next 18 months all direct frontline staff will have been trained in the Patient First system (more on that to come), working ward by ward in a four-module programme which includes a lot of leadership coaching in between more formal sessions. Supporting the capability development is the second foundation, or Kaizen Office, a team of skilled people who help to pull it all together, support and coach local teams. The Kaizen Office also supports the third foundation of Priority Initiatives. These are a small number of chosen bigger initiatives, such as using Lean to improve our stroke pathway.

And, most importantly, our work does not stop here. I mentioned earlier that we were determined to bring together improvement functions and efforts *and* management systems and processes. We held a shared belief, and still do, that the reason why Lean sometimes doesn't stick is that it can become, and be viewed as, a basketful of projects. From the outset, Helen and the rest of us on the board have been adamant that this is not just a project: improvement is our work. This is the way we are going to run our organisation. Thankfully, the wind has been in our favour. There had not been earlier failed attempts to introduce Lean, and Helen and her team had built up fabulous goodwill in the organisation. She was trusted. I would go as far as to say that she was, and still is, loved in the organisation. And still, there was some cynicism in the early days:

"Here's another improvement project, another project that we're going to go through that people will lose interest in, but if we keep our heads down it will be OK."

And so, to ensure that this way of working was to be more than just our rhetoric, we made two further moves, adding two further foundations. The first was to introduce, develop and refine our Patient First Improvement System based upon Lean principles. The second was to make patient care and improvement central to our strategy and our strategy deployment.

The Patient First system is a Lean system and way of working that supports and enables our local ward and unit teams to deliver improvement. This includes what you might expect of a Lean-informed system. For example, we have local daily improvement huddles, at 8.30 and midday; we use both PDSA and A3 Thinking as approaches to structured problem solving, and have some fantastic visual management. I lead on this aspect and am particularly proud of how we have evolved and improved the system from the experience and learning of the teams using it. It looks quite different today compared with how we started out.

For example, in the early days we introduced the idea of a ward "daily status sheet conversation". This is a tool that one of our partners uses to good effect. However, for us, this idea didn't work. We already had safety huddles well-embedded in the wards. These are short conversations at the beginning of every day that ask five key questions and involve all staff, not just the senior nurses. We found ourselves doing both, having the safety huddles and then the status sheet conversations. Staff soon pushed back:

"You talk about Lean? This isn't Lean!"

We persevered for a while and then reflected that the status sheet conversations, as well as duplicating effort, were a bit too transactional and excluding for our culture. It felt more honest for us and our culture to stay with the safety huddles, involving everyone from the ward teams. We have dropped the status sheet conversations in the wards.

I try and go to three or four improvement huddles a week. Not because I want to direct but because I want to listen and understand the problems and the opportunities for improvement. Sometimes I will coach a bit, ask questions, be curious. If I had to choose the biggest thing we can do as leaders to foster improvement it would be to ask curious questions. It engages people, uncovers all sorts of stuff and opens up possibilities. And I would say, almost as strongly, genuine intention to be useful is also vital. This idea of visible leadership, to show up to be seen on the wards, is just nonsense to me and can get in the way of the work. If you show up as a leader there needs to be a purpose, a purpose to listen, understand and offer support as is needed.

In the early days of each improvement huddle we are careful about how we show up – all the exec team join the huddles as part of our agreed standard work. When they are starting out, some can be nervous that if we show up, they are on show, facing a bit of scrutiny. We take great pains to signal that we are there to support and observe and not to judge. If there are any performance issues, we *never* raise them in the huddles. Similarly, we never challenge or criticise in public. Staff need to know that the huddles are safe and developmental, that they will not be made to feel awkward, or shamed. As the huddles mature and become more experienced, we find staff want to use them as opportunities to share what they are proud of, and even junior members of staff jostle to have the opportunity to take the lead, and to shine.

And the Patient First system is working. So many ward teams in the NHS today feel ground down with layer upon layer of demand. And that is where we were, with ward staff confiding in me that they didn't know for how long they could go on. Now, the mood and energy has shifted. Staff know what the priorities are, and they know that they can make a difference. They have also experienced how this way of working can release time to care.

Finally, our strategy foundation. If I am honest, I don't think as leaders in the NHS we are very good at strategy. Most of what we do is about financial management, and we can be very reluctant to make choices and say no, and yet, as Peter Block says (2007), "If we cannot say 'no' then our 'yes' has no meaning." Our strategy is simple and can be encapsulated in one page. At the core is the focus on quality of patient care, and quality improvement as the means to deliver it. We have six three-to-five-year organisation objectives or priorities, each with a very small number of carefully chosen but straight forward metrics to guide us. We call these our "True North" objectives, and avoiding harm, mentioned earlier, is one. It's not rocket science, but as an exec team we have not been ashamed to say throughout the organisation that this is what we have decided our organisation success will look like. Even though as a team we are committed to facilitating and coaching, at times it is appropriate to demonstrate leadership and set direction.

It was a salutary lesson for us when we sat down to choose the objectives. We began by listing out all ongoing strategic initiatives and corporate projects. There were hundreds, literally hundreds. The rigour we had to go through to select just six objectives was hard. It was real learning for us to have to choose and say "No, we are not going to do that". It was a good experience to help us be more empathetic and useful to our ward and unit teams when we asked them to choose. More on that next.

As well as guiding resource allocation (time and money) and performance management at board level, our strategy and objectives guide our wards and units in prioritising local improvement initiatives. We used to be spread a mile wide and an inch deep, and it was near impossible to be able to see any progress. If everything is a priority, then nothing is a priority. So my mantra to our teams now is to focus more, to be an inch wide and a mile deep. All teams, as part of the Patient First system, generate "improvement tickets" for improvements they identify. They are like gold dust – rather like the golden tickets in *Charlie and the Chocolate Factory* – and we measure the number to encourage people to come forward. And yet, each of the wards and units have, at any time, only three "just do its" and three PDSA improvement tickets ongoing. The rest can wait in a queue. The teams make their own decisions about which tickets to prioritise based on real data, their A3 sheets and ultimately, the strategic question of whether and how does the proposed improvement move us forward against one or more of the objectives. Imagine the sense of ownership this creates as well as momentum for improvement, every day, across the organisation.

I am feeling concern that I might be making this sound too easy and a recipe for others to follow. My hope is that our story can encourage others to believe they can find a similar story of their own, one that works for their culture, trusting that it can work. Personally, I have never doubted that it can work, nor looked back with any regret. Perhaps too it has been more straightforward than we might even have dreamed of. The good starting point certainly made a difference. And yet, there have been times of real challenge, as well as more personal "dark night of the soul" moments for me.

I have faced a couple of big tests. Early on I had to deal with some difficult medics, consultants whose self-interests and values were at odds with what we wanted to do and how we wanted to be as an organisation. I knew that I had Helen and the Chairman's support, but it still took a few frank and honest conversations at the end of which a small but not insignificant number of consultants left the organisation. I like to think of myself as quite a gentle soul and my personal drivers mean that conflict and disharmony are not things I welcome. I have standards and a strong sense of moral values though, and these give me the courage to stand firm when I need to, and don't allow me to avoid the difficult stuff.

A more personally distressing event was when, in the midst of things going well, the exec team was accused by a whistle-blower of being bullying, discriminatory and acting with self-interest rather than the interests of patients. Helen and I were named individually and singled out as being particularly at fault. This could not have come at a worse time, just before a CQC inspection, and out of the blue we went from being tucked away and out of sight to having red flags waving from every building, metaphorically that is. The CQC were on it instantly, "What's going on down there?", as were the GMC and our local MP.

Helen and I did a lot of soul searching. The accusations touched us both deeply. We began to doubt whether we were seeing ourselves properly. We thought that we were perceived as kind and supportive and doing the right thing – things that matter to both of us – but we began to wonder whether we had got it wrong and that was not how we were perceived at all. It was tough.

This was a time when the teamwork amongst the execs really mattered and the relationships we have with each other held us firm, and kept us psychologically safe. Together, we got to the place of realising that we had to respond, to hear the accusation and investigate. We couldn't investigate it internally as we were all involved, so we had to bring in an external investigator. None of the allegations was found to be true but it was a really damaging time, and it cost the CQC a lot of anxiety too. When they came to do the inspection, they had additional, special meetings to explore allegations of bullying and to question our leadership capability. I can remember feeling confident, and yet troublingly vulnerable at the same time. It was a horrible time; one where your values are scrutinised and questioned, and one of those times when you have to take a good long look at yourself.

There were bright sides in all of this, however. Most of my consultant colleagues were copied in to the allegations, and 70 or so chose to write independently to the CQC ahead of the inspection. They were outraged that a colleague could do this, not just personally to the exec team but to *their* organisation. A lot of positive feedback came our way from this, as well as a real sense that we were well supported. When the CQC held their focus groups they had to open up more rooms, as too many people wanted to come and tell them what they are proud of and the things we are good at. One of the lead inspectors was heard to say:

"I've got half an hour, it's great but I really have to ask is nobody going to say something negative about this organisation?"

So I am coming not to the end of the story, as we still have a lot to do, but to a pause. Together, as an organisation, we have achieved a lot. The CQC rated us as outstanding, which is a nice badge to have; but more important than that is the improvement in care we are now achieving for our patients. We are now fourth in the country as measured by A&E targets, are fully compliant against all seven cancer metrics and are in the top quartile of Trusts nationally for mortality figures. We also have steadily improving staff engagement feedback. I haven't mentioned money much in this story, if at all, but we have also managed to pay back more than £20 million of legacy debt. Our challenge now is not to become complacent, to keep on our toes, to hold on to a sense of humility and, for the exec team, to avoid the trap of group-think.

I was asked recently what did I think had contributed most to the apparent success in this story. When I reflected on my response I was interested to realise that I didn't mention Lean once, although I have no doubt that the good use of this approach and the underlying philosophy has had enormous benefit. What I did mention was consistency of leadership, which is rare indeed now in the NHS. I also mentioned paying attention to relationships and the culture that follows from that. I see my role, and I know Helen does too, about primarily forming good relationships throughout the organisation and I hope that is evident in the story. We use every possible means to connect with people, whether with teams, with individuals, face to face or even via Twitter and WhatsApp! If you don't have good relationships with people, how do you develop trust and how can you expect people to follow you?

Returning to the beginning of this story and the question of why I couldn't do what I wanted to do in my previous organisation, I think it's about two things: power and context. The reality is I now have sufficient positional power, as a member of the board, to make and inform strategic decisions on behalf of the organisation. I have both the freedom and the accountability with my board colleagues to steer a course. We also have a sense of space and time to follow through. In the NHS, too often we are obsessed with turnaround and quick fixes, and when the fix doesn't happen fast enough we change the leadership team. To me, it's a form of madness; madness which so far we have been protected from by stable leadership, acceptable financial performance and good quality indicators – all of which every team in the organisation continues to work hard to maintain and improve.

I was also asked whether I miss clinical practice. I haven't practised medicine now for some five years. I want to do a really good job in whatever I do and reached the conclusion that I could not do both, practise clinically and be a medical director. Yet, I still think of myself as a clinician and take the time to talk shop with my medical colleagues. It is an important part of my identity. My work is to improve patient care, so whether I do that by fixing someone in theatre or by improving the system it doesn't really matter. Both are ultimately about patients.

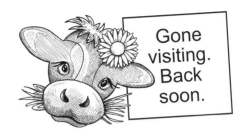

CHAPTER 13

Daisy

Daisy is a small pink fibreglass cow. To be precise, she is more a calf than a cow.

She began life in a local shopping centre as an advertising aid, but now lives in a glass display cabinet on the main corridor of a children's hospital where she visibly promotes and celebrates patient safety and quality improvement initiatives. This is her story as much as mine. It's a story I never imagined I would be telling. It's an example of what can happen when you make a simple gesture as a leader, a gesture which is different and is noticed and amplified by others. It shows what can happen when people working together on something important allow themselves to have some fun alongside the very serious business of caring for patients, and it shows the power of an idea to create energy and momentum for quality improvement.

To start, I need to take you back to when I joined the department over 12 years ago. I had successfully completed my training and had been appointed to a post in a department that I had worked in as a registrar. I expected my transition to consultant to be easy. It therefore came as a great shock to me when I felt frustration and isolation such as I had never experienced before. Initially I attributed these feelings to the fact that I was the only female in the department, was new to the role, and was less experienced than the others. It took me a long time to realise that what I was experiencing had less to do with me as an individual and more to do with the departmental culture.

What I did not appreciate then is that because my new colleagues had been working together for many years, they had shared significant history, had learned how to relate easily to each other and had established norms of behaviour. I did not realise that the arrival of anyone new, including me, was always going to challenge the status quo of the existing culture within the group.

This situation was made more difficult by the fact that, prior to my appointment, the department had been involved in an inquiry into patient care. When they spoke about this difficult time, I noticed that many colleagues felt they had been inadequately supported. The inquiry had cast a long shadow over everyone. Consequently, and understandably, they had become somewhat professionally defensive, appearing risk averse and suspicious of others' motives. It appeared to me that an unintended conse-quence of the inquiry was that my consultant colleagues were reluctant to offer me, and at times each other, any support. If I asked a colleague for a view in relation to something to do with a patient's care, there often seemed to be reluctance on their part to offer a response, to say what they would do. The sense I made of this at the time was that they were fearful that if I were later criticised for what I had done, then they too, by association, would also be criticised. I felt that I had joined a department where the dominant culture appeared to be one of fear and blame.

What kept me going during this time was my enduring desire to look after sick children. I developed strong working relationships with my nursing colleagues and slowly began to feel I belonged. The department also gradually increased in size, and I now have several female colleagues and colleagues of different nationalities. What had felt like an insular culture now feels as if it has shifted to be one that is more inviting and more accepting of difference.

A turning point came for me after a near miss, an episode that could so easily have developed to become a critical incident. Feeling very isolated during this time, I decided to become involved in clinical governance to learn more about how to manage adverse patient incidents and to build my own support network. It was through this that I became really interested in quality improvement and spotted an opportunity to gain a Scottish Patient Safety Programme (SPSP) Fellowship. As part of being on this programme, I was required to initiate a quality improvement project in my own area.

"If you're not sure what you want to improve, think about what bugs you on a Monday morning!" the tutor said to us all.

What was bugging me on a Monday morning was the minimal focus on operational and safety issues. We carried out a formal sit-down systematic clinical review of each patient's care at the morning handover in the PICU unit seminar room, and we would talk about how patients were progressing clinically, what medication they currently required, what investigations were needed. We would then go round the beds and actually see the patients, and it was often only at that point that one of the nurses, or maybe a junior doctor, would speak up and say,

"Do you know we nearly had a drug error last night?" or

"This patient is going to the MRI scanner this afternoon," or

"This piece of equipment gave us trouble overnight".

In order to try to increase focus on issues like these, I decided that my project for the SPSP Fellowship would be centred on increasing staff awareness of safety and quality issues within the Paediatric Intensive Care Unit (PICU) through a daily PICU multidisciplinary team (MDT) safety brief.

My idea was to have a five-minute safety brief, in the form of a conversation with as many staff as possible, about any actual or potential safety issues, and that the brief would occur just before the systematic review. I identified a number of staff from the PICU MDT and formed a safety brief project group. Together we devised a simple checklist to use during the safety brief. The checklist consisted of short questions such as: How many patients are in the unit? Are there any empty beds? Any issues relating to staffing levels, infection control, equipment, medication, near misses, and so on? The methodology we used for this project was the Model for Improvement, and our aim was that within six months of starting the project, a daily multidisciplinary safety brief would occur on at least on at 95 percent of mornings per month.

I decided to invite everyone to the safety brief: physiotherapists, technicians, consultants, junior doctors, pharmacists, senior nurses, junior nurses, students, clerical staff and domestic staff. To encourage attendance, I spoke personally with as many staff as I could, as well as sending emails. The message was the same – everyone was welcome, please come and add anything they felt should be included.

The invitation went down well, and the topics brought for discussion and inclusion on the checklist began to evolve. Feedback from staff was that the questions asked on the checklist were really helpful. For instance, asking about bed occupancy was important because, while there may be a free bed in a two-bedded area, it may not be possible to use this free bed depending on infection control issues. Clarifying these issues early in the morning meant that communication was improved, as was planning.

I had no idea about the impact this invitation would have in terms of getting everyone involved. In fact, a general theme of my story is that I am continually surprised at what emerges from quite simple gestures when others feel included and empowered to add and act upon their own ideas.

One of the main challenge to implementing the safety brief was the way we consultants worked within PICU. There was little sense of team or ongoing relationships. While there is no doubt that we were all trying to do the very best for our patients, we didn't have anything that brought this all together. If, for example, I was on duty in PICU on a Monday but then in theatre for the rest of the week, the rest of the PICU team had to work with a different duty consultant on other days, each with potentially different views and priorities. I believed that introducing a safety brief would improve team work and communication, but I was worried that the safety brief would happen only when I was on duty in PICU – and not when I wasn't!

To try to get the safety brief off the ground, I decided that I would do the brief myself every Monday for about four weeks and not worry about what happened on the other days. Then I would pop in every other day, saying to my consultant colleagues in theatre, "Just going to do the safety brief." "OK," they would reply, looking a bit askance.

To my delight, what started happening was that even on the days when I was not on duty in PICU, the junior doctors and the nurses insisted that they wanted to do the safety brief. They would come to the morning handover with the safety brief checklist in their hand, ready to use, so it was hard then for my consultant colleagues to ignore their request and their enthusiasm.

As the brief involved the use of a paper-based checklist, I decided to keep copies of it in an A4 folder that I had found lying around at home. It was colourful, so stood out from the plain office-grey ones. Despite the folder, I learned that on days when the brief didn't happen, one of the reasons given was that staff could not find a copy of the checklist.

I looked closely at the A4 folder and happened to notice that it was adorned with brightly coloured cows. Looking back now at what some might call an act of madness, or trivia, I decided to put a fun image of a cow on every piece of paperwork associated with the safety brief. Trivial or not, it worked. Using the image in this way proved to be a very effective way of engaging staff and helping them to remember to do the safety brief.

One of the nurses decided we needed a whiteboard to record key items emerging from the brief. She found the money from somewhere to secure a board and personally wrote on it the aim: to achieve a daily multidisciplinary safety brief on at least 95 percent of mornings within the next six months.

One of my consultant colleagues wanted to know how we were going to measure this, so we created something that was a bit like a children's rota that you might have on your fridge at home, with names and coloured dots for the different professional groups – blue for pharmacy, orange for nurses, green for the physiotherapists, red for junior doctors and so on. This "safety brief staff attendance wall chart" was displayed in the PICU seminar room for all staff to see. The chart created a bit of fun and some competition, and yet real data began to emerge. One of the junior doctors commented that there was always a dip in attendance at the safety brief on a Thursday. A consultant colleague was heard to say "Blow this. I am not going to be having a dip on my day", so he started doing the safety brief and encouraging all staff to attend. Participation had now begun to improve – especially on a Thursday!

Many staff commented that through the brief they felt empowered to raise safety issues which they would otherwise not have raised, as it was an environment where everyone's concerns were listened to. The safety brief also gave staff an opportunity to come together, at a designated time, every day, to identify, share and communicate safety concerns, so we had created a supportive and learning environment for everyone, without fear and blame.

I began to notice something else. We were focusing on safety and ways to improve quality of care in the discussions at the safety brief, and yet we were also having fun, smiling and thinking of other ways we could use our cow image. Nursing colleagues decided to put the cow image on the safety brief staff attendance wall chart. They also put the image on a notice which they placed at the nurses' station inviting all staff to attend the brief. The cow was becoming a member of the team in a way I hadn't expected. And the cow started changing the atmosphere on the unit, bringing us together and creating a little bit of fun.

As the weeks passed it was clear that we were going to achieve our aim, to have implemented a daily safety brief on 95 percent of mornings per month. Realising how significant this achievement was, I wanted to celebrate this success with the PICU team. I thought about making a cake. I thought about buying balloons. And yet I was so proud of everyone, I really wanted to do something different and special. Around this time one of the nurses, Susan, joked and laughed with me about the number of cow images appearing in PICU. "I wouldn't be surprised if I walked into PICU one day and saw a real cow!" she said.

Her comment stuck in my head.

A few days later, when I was in a local shopping mall, I noticed a number of fibreglass cows on display. They were being used to collect money for charity and were all coloured pink to celebrate the first stage of the Giro d'Italia cycling event, which was beginning in the city that year. I was reminded of my recent conversation with Susan and began to imagine how much fun it would be if I could rent or borrow one of these cows, just for a day, and bring it to PICU to celebrate the success of the safety brief. As well as celebrating the success of the brief, I began to realise that Daisy – as she later became affectionately known – represented more than the successful implementation of the safety brief, she also represented the seemingly impossible becoming possible (like finding a cow in PICU!). I was thrilled at the way a seemingly random idea could come to life and effect change.

So nervously, and yet excitedly, I made inquiries and spoke with the manager of the shopping centre, fully expecting him to think my idea for this celebration was crazy.

"Could you tell me how much your cows are?" I said. "Or could I rent one for a couple of hours?"

I explained about the safety brief and the children's hospital. He was enthusiastic:

"It's a great idea. How many do you want? You can have them for free."

"Oh my goodness. Are you for real?" I couldn't believe he wasn't laughing at me and was convinced it was a great idea.

It was a challenge getting the cow, who was now white again, into the back of my car as, being made of fibreglass, she was rather rigid. Ears, legs, tail, they wouldn't budge, but eventually my husband and I managed to squeeze her onto the back seat of the car. You can probably imagine the looks on the faces of passers-by. On a Sunday evening, we crept into the hospital together, cow hidden under a blanket, and placed her in the PICU seminar room. At 9.00am on Monday morning, there she was, in all her glory. And it was nothing but laughter:

"What are we going to do with the cow?"

"Can we have a photograph taken with the cow?"

"Can we paint her?"

"Can we name her?"

Someone called out, "Daisy," and that's what stuck. I left the staff to decide on the colour. They wanted to paint her pink again, with little daisies on her back.

The arrival of Daisy provoked so many conversations: "What's this with the cow?" "Why's she here?"

We explained about the safety brief and our good work and the chart, and people started to get really interested. But we ran into problems. Due to strict infection control, Daisy could not stay in PICU, and so we had to find somewhere else to put her. I spotted a glass display cabinet on the main corridor of the hospital. I asked the service manager about it. He had plans to install an antique rocking horse, but I asked whether Daisy could go there instead. He shrugged his shoulders, "You can try, but I doubt she'll fit."

But I knew if I could squeeze her into my car that this was no challenge, and she is still there today; and to explain why she was there, we placed a sign on the cabinet that said,

"Congratulations PICU, Safety Brief Success!"

Whilst initially disappointed that Daisy could not stay in PICU, locating Daisy in this cabinet resulted in further unexpected success. Staff from other areas of the hospital were curious and began asking about the safety brief and what Daisy represented. They decided they too would like to implement a safety brief, and so Daisy helped to spread the success of the safety brief beyond PICU and to begin conversations about safety and quality improvement. Other QI initiatives began, not only in the children's hospital but also throughout the main hospital.

Later in the year, a senior director asked if Daisy could help support the launch of a new Trust-wide Patient Safety and QI campaign. This campaign involves using the Trust intranet as a platform on which staff from across the organisation can celebrate and share their QI initiatives. Daisy was delighted to help with the launch of this inaugural campaign, and has continued to support this campaign every year since. Through the campaign Daisy is now instantly recognisable across the whole hospital – maybe for some staff she is more recognisable than the executive team!

As part of the campaign Daisy was invited to visit a number of areas across the organisation. One such invitation was from a group of adults with learning needs, based in the community. This group wanted to meet Daisy and to have their photo taken with her. They wanted this photo to be featured as a hospital intranet news story, in order to highlight how they too were focusing on safety and quality. Daisy helped them to feel part of the organisation and gave focus to their good work.

So occasionally Daisy has travelled to various events across the organisation, to help promote and celebrate safety and quality improvement. However, people in the children's hospital started to become worried about where Daisy was if she wasn't in her display cabinet, so we had signs printed that said, "Just away for today – to the Chief Executive's briefing," or wherever else she had gone visiting that day.

And Daisy now has a guardian: a good friend of mine who works in theatres has the key to the display cabinet, and now manages Daisy's diary.

The hospital went on to launch their staff eight-month QI training programme. Daisy was asked to support this programme. Successful participants were given a Daisy badge to wear to symbolise their support for QI. Through this programme many participants subsequently used Daisy's image to help implement QI projects in their local area.

Daisy has become a very important member of the PICU team and the children's hospital. Her presence has become a catalyst for many QI initiatives, including:

1. *"What matters to me?"* This patient-centred initiative involves using a bedside card on which a child or parent can write what matters to their child, what kind of things would help to make their stay in PICU better. The name of the child's favourite toy, their pet dog, their favourite song are often written on these cards. Daisy also appears on these cards, visibly endorsing this initiative as an important piece of QI.

2. *Daily goals in PICU.* As there had been recent evidence in the literature that the use of daily goals in the intensive care setting could lead to improvement in quality of patient care, the PICU team decided to devise a daily goals checklist. In order to get staff buy-in, one of my consultant colleagues devised a checklist framed around the mnemonic "BFFDAISY", where BFF is a play on the common digital form of affection "Best Forever Friend". Each letter of "BFFDAISY" represents a key area of patient care in PICU: B = Blood results, F= Fluids, F=Food, D=Medication A=alerts I= Infection control S= sedation Y = what is the indication for on-going intensive care (that is to say, should we now be planning for discharge)? Some of the PICU team submitted a poster describing this initiative to a medical conference and chose the title "Safety and Quality through Friendship in PICU ".

3. *The "ZAP the VAP" initiative.* The PICU team wanted to implement the use of a "High Impact Care Bundle" in PICU. They wanted to implement the care bundle associated with reducing the incidence of Ventilator-Associated Pneumonia or "VAP".

   To engage staff in the implementation of this care bundle, some of the PICU team decided that they would like to re-create Daisy as a super-hero. So Daisy wore a mask and cape for a few weeks to raise the profile of this initiative. Her cape was adorned with the motto "ZAP the VAP"!

4. *Changing from hand-written to electronic post-operative surgical notes.*
   One of the surgeons wanted to lead a QI intuitive to change practice from hand-written post-operative surgical notes to electronic notes. The surgeon called me up and asked for Daisy's help to promote this change in practice. "Daisy is delighted to be invited," I said, and on the day that this initiative was being launched, we took Daisy out of her display cabinet and placed her on the main theatre corridor with an accompanying sign describing the initiative. The surgeon sent me some lovely photos of himself and three nurses with Daisy, all grinning away, promoting this initiative.

5. *Antibiotic Stewardship.* Daisy was asked to support a campaign to highlight the importance of appropriate use of antibiotics. Again, I replied that she was thrilled, feeling that I had rather become like Daisy's agent. The staff leading on this initiative placed posters it beside Daisy and on her display cabinet. Because of the location of Daisy in her cabinet on the main corridor in the children's hospital, all staff knew that, as a hospital, we were taking part in "Antibiotic Stewardship week".

6. *"Learning from Excellence" initiative.* Staff from PICU and from the Emergency Department recently introduced an IR2 or "Learning from Excellence" award. With much emphasis on reporting adverse incidents via an Incident Report, or "IR1", these staff decided to create an "IR2" whereby staff can nominate any member of staff within the children's hospital who they feel deserves recognition for their good work. The award is a certificate endorsed and signed by Daisy. This initiative won a recent Trust-wide Chairman's award, and both the award and photos of staff celebrating receiving it were placed on Daisy's cabinet for a few weeks – to visibly share this success with all staff within the Trust.

7. *Daisy as compassion.* Staff in PICU love Daisy and what she represents so much, that they decided see if they could get a soft toy replica of Daisy made to order. So we now have a Daisy soft toy (a pink cow with a daisy flower on her head), that we give to all families in PICU as way of expressing compassion to children and their families during their stay, and to share our passion to put safety and quality at the centre of our clinical care.

8. *Daisy as a brand.* As the story of Daisy's impact on QI grew, staff wanted to develop a Daisy image that they could use to endorse QI and QI initiatives. A photo of her in her glass display cabinet was felt to be inadequate, and so a Trust-based graphic designer helped us to create a cute image of Daisy.

Because of the success of Daisy and how proud the staff in the children's hospital are of their QI initiatives to date, one of the service managers decided to use this cute image of Daisy to get pink Daisy lanyards made and Daisy badges that all staff can wear, and many do wear, to symbolise their support for QI and to create a sense of pride in the Trust. Just the other day I saw one of our very alpha male consultants wearing his Daisy lanyard with pride. She has brought huge organisational recognition to QI and to the hospital, which is a significant achievement given the enormous size and complexity of the organisation.

For me, Daisy represents the successful use of an artefact in helping to promote a culture of safety and quality improvement. Through Daisy we have been able to work better as a team, a department, and maybe even as an organisation, and she has given us moments of great joy at work. Even though I did not realise it at the time, Daisy has allowed me to re-connect with my creative side. Because of her success in engaging staff in QI, Daisy has somehow also given other staff permission to release their creativity, with amazing results. Daisy has helped create an environment where staff have become empowered to come up with their own ideas for improvement and to test these ideas on a small scale in their local area.

To me she also represents possibility, the possibility that what may seem as a daft idea may not be daft at all, and just might be an idea that is highly effective in bringing about change and improvement, not just at a local level but perhaps elsewhere in the organisation, and maybe even across the health care system. So, to me, she also represents excitement and the possibility of bottom-up change.

She has brought an element of fun and playfulness into clinical environments that are highly intense and emotionally draining – most notably PICU. Through her, the staff in PICU are constantly seeking out new ways of improving. She has brought a sense of pride to PICU and helped to develop a spirit of collaboration.

I am also not blind to the fact that there are many staff who do not like Daisy. They don't see her as relevant. They don't like the cow image, and many have declared their dislike of the colour pink. Some will openly say, "Not that cow again," but that's OK. Other people do want her, and she doesn't need to be liked by everyone.

I have learned from Daisy too. I have learned that it is not necessary for everyone to love and appreciate Daisy for her to be effective in creating a culture of safety and quality. Neither is it necessary for everyone to love me for me to lead effectively. This has been particularly liberating for me in my leadership, given that I now realise that one of my strongest personal drivers is one to Please People.

I have also realised that for creativity and innovation to emerge it is good to have diversity. When I discuss the story of Daisy with those who do not love her, or perhaps even like her, I realise now that these discussions are a form of engagement, a conversation that may never have taken place without having the concept of Daisy to debate. Like Daisy or loathe Daisy, subliminally she has been the catalyst for beginning many conversations around safety and quality, for exploring the possibilities of improvement.

And often when I look back at all that Daisy has achieved so far, and I think of all the plans we have for using her to continue to create a culture of continuous improvement and to create joy at work, I wonder if Daisy's story is really my story.

Through Daisy, I know that I have developed courage to lead in ways that I would never had thought possible before. The QI initiatives that my colleagues and friends in the children's hospital and the wider organisation have led on, and the way they have used Daisy to endorse and promote these initiatives, have made my heart sing and my feet dance. As I write this I feel that for Daisy (and for me) there is much, much, more to come!

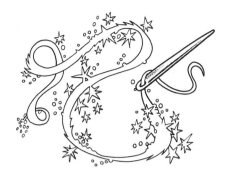

CHAPTER 14

The Thread of Kindness

There's a lovely Chinese proverb which suggests that as leaders we can't really make anything happen – all we can do is create a space in which what we want is more likely to happen.

I look around my organisation now and I consider myself to be in a very fortunate and privileged position: my role as Director of Patient Experience has influence, and was the first of its kind in the NHS. It has given me some of the most rewarding work of my career to date.

According to staff survey results, the colleagues I work with are consistently rated as being amongst the most engaged NHS staff in the country. The risk my board took eight years ago to innovate and invest in understanding and improving patient experience has paid off handsomely.

The latest national inpatient patient experience results published last month show that the Trust has moved from a ranking position of 111th in 2009 to 11th in 2017, the best non-specialist organisation in the country. During this time, the focus of our organisation has clearly changed: 86 percent of our staff now believe that high-quality patient care is the number one priority of the Trust, whereas previously it had been only 43 percent.

As I reflect on these achievements, I am aware of both a sense of pride and deep gratitude for the fertile ground that made change possible. In this chapter, I want to explore what it is about my organisation that encouraged and enabled some of my very early improvement ideas to take root and grow.

As I wind the clock back I'm also curious – if I was starting this work all over again, would I be given the same freedom and opportunities in 2017 that I was trusted with in 2009? Would I also take the same approach with the increased knowledge and experience that I have now?

A new role

Eight years ago, I was working late on the Stroke Unit one evening and I decided to read the latest Don Berwick publication on person-centred care. The paper was entitled *Confessions of an Extremist* and in it he outlined exactly why he feared becoming a patient:

> ......*to be made helpless before my time, to be made ignorant when I want to know, to be made to sit when I wish to stand, to be alone when I need to hold my wife's hand, to eat what I do not wish to eat, to be named what I do not wish to be named, to be told when I wish to be asked, to be awoken when I wish to sleep.*

(Berwick 2009)

He spoke of dreading the anonymity and powerlessness of the hospital gown and why he believed the needs of institutions will always trump the needs of the individual. His words touched me deeply and I had to admit that when I looked around the institution in which I worked, I recognised that all of his fears had substance. I felt troubled and unnerved by the words I had read. I also felt ashamed. I could see that that we weren't doing enough to listen to patients and understand more about their own views, personal values and choices.

The paper invited me to embrace and promote the type of care that encourages individuals to assert their humanity and their individuality. I felt compelled to take up that challenge. Without thinking too hard, I contacted my Chief Executive, Medical Director, and Business Unit Director for Medicine and Emergency Care, sending them a copy of the paper with a post-it note saying "What are we doing to promote person-centred care in this organisation? "

When I have shared this story in the past, some people have found it hard to believe that senior leaders took me seriously and responded in the way they did, so I tell this story because I believe it reveals important elements about the organisation in which I work and my relationship to it. Firstly, something about the organisational culture must have told me that it was OK to invite this discussion with the senior leaders. Secondly, whilst I knew the action wasn't completely without reputational risk, I certainly wasn't inhibited from speaking up or approaching executive colleagues by a rigid sense of hierarchy and control. They felt near enough to me to approach and open enough to welcome new ideas.

Whilst national staff survey results suggest that people in my organisation do indeed feel very comfortable about raising concerns, I'm aware that what the Trust doesn't appear to tolerate very well is folk moaning about problems from the side-lines. So if you raise a quality issue expect to be listened to, but also expect to be given responsibility for helping to make things better.

And so it was with me. The final outcome of a number of conversations about person-centred care was a new job: I was appointed as Director of Patient Experience in December 2009.

As I reflect on this now, I'm curious as to what it was about me that made this new post feel like such a neat fit? The new opportunity emerged in a climate of trust: the faith I'd shown in my organisation and senior leaders by speaking up was rewarded and also returned by their faith in me. I was given freedom to experiment, time to explore, and respect to design the compassionate improvement programme that I wanted.

In those very early days, it was wonderful to discover that I could rely on strong and continued support from the board, and the CEO and Chairman in particular. I recognise now what an exceptional gift this was.

Although exciting and new in 2009, my expectation would be that directors of patient experience would now be routinely found on Trust boards in 2017. Sadly, the nature of my role, the level of autonomy given, and the specific responsibility to improve patient experience alone, has not been replicated since in another NHS organisation. Instead patient experience is a remit that competes with many others in a squeezed and pressured exec director portfolio.

I believe that this speaks volumes about the relative importance given to patient experience compared to other more externally focused issues like performance or finance in the current NHS landscape.

Understanding what matters

In the summer before taking up my new role, I was on holiday with my family in a very rural part of Turkey. On our final day, I persuaded my husband to leave our children with their grandparents by the pool, whilst we hired a couple of motorbikes and headed to the hills.

It didn't end well, I lost control of my bike, collided with a fruit lorry and was transported away, unconscious.

It is still very hard to describe just how frightened I was to wake up in the back of an old ambulance in a strange country. All of my innate prejudices came to the fore; there was no part of me that believed that I was about to receive high-quality, safe and effective health care.

I was transferred to the nearest hospital which happened to be a brand new, sparkling clean building that had been open for less than three weeks.

My initial assessment was thorough with rapid access to CT scanning, and the results immediately shared by a considerate and friendly consultant. On transfer to HDU there was no shortage of attention from five nurses who were desperate to care for someone...anyone!

All objective indicators of safety and quality were clearly evident to me, and yet I was too frightened to trust – I just wanted to be back in the UK.

That night a young man came to see me; he explained that he worked on reception downstairs, he said had no medical knowledge but that he had previously worked in the hospitality industry. He said he imagined that I was very frightened, he knew I was a long way from home, and he wanted to help.

He offered the gift of his excellent English; he said he would come and visit me every day, and if there were questions I wanted to ask the health care team he would ask them on my behalf.

His kindness that night had a profound impact. I relaxed, began to trust the team and recovered well. I returned to my new job with an even deeper commitment to understand more about the things that *really* matter to people when they're lying frightened in our hospital beds.

Measuring what matters

The early months of joining the executive management team felt quite difficult for me. I really missed working with patients and families every day; I missed the familiar buzz of the ward environment, and the warmth of the stroke family that I'd been part of for more than 15 years. As a consultant speech and language therapist I was used to influencing practice and decision-making within the multidisciplinary team. I enjoyed teaching and developing others and I felt confident about my level of knowledge and competence within this particular specialty.

In the new corporate environment, I felt awkward, uncomfortable and lonely; I'd never worn suits, and my aspiration to just make things better for patients at times felt hopelessly naïve. In debates over resources I would listen to people demanding "hard" facts on one matter or another, and became convinced that my own credibility depended on developing a robust measurement framework on which to evidence change.

I wanted reliable intelligence on patient experience at my fingertips as I sat beside more powerful and influential colleagues. I look back now and recognise that perhaps this insecurity has served me well. I'm very proud of the person-centred metrics that underpin our patient experience programme, and the fact that it is recognised as one of the most developed and robust measurement frameworks in the NHS.

We capture the views of 50,000 people every year and we do this in a variety of ways; this enables me to provide real-time information on performance at every level of the Trust. I can, for example, demonstrate how my organisation has improved year on year. I was able to report on the impact of our new emergency care hospital according to the views of the first 1,000 people through the doors. We can trace the difference of experience within a particular specialty – the difference between trauma and an elective surgical experience for example – and also understand the variation in care and compassion that exists on every ward and between individual consultants.

As someone who loves data, this granular understanding of my own organisation excites and motivates me. The support from the board has been critical, and yet it's the way the programme has engaged staff that I am perhaps most proud of.

In true QI style, my first tests of real-time measurement were deliberately modest. As a small team of three we chose to visit eight wards across two hospital sites every fortnight. We'd speak to as many people as we could, at least 50 percent of those present on the ward each time, gathering data and facilitating connections between the needs of patients and the response from staff.

Within six months we saw the statistical benefit of real-time improvement. Our programme had also attracted the attention of others: we received many calls asking if the patient experience programme would be coming to their ward anytime soon.

At this point, I resisted pressure from the board to roll out real-time measurement, everywhere, and at pace. I'm glad I did – a slower, more considered, incremental roll out allowed us to support and spend time with teams in the process of improving, as well as listen to their excellent ideas for change.

The programme has enabled us to shine a light on interactions. I now believe that simply paying attention, noticing and giving staff regular feedback, good or bad, is an act of kindness in itself. People deserve to be appreciated for all they are getting right and they deserve to feel quickly and appropriately supported to improve when standards fall short.

For me it's not a question of "hard" data or "subjective" stories – we need both. Routine measurement and regular conversations with patients and families have revealed beautiful examples of care at its very best. I've found hope in the discovery of many everyday heroes, and the incredible kindness that exists in the NHS despite the pressure, noise and complexity of delivering health care.

I've witnessed times when the emotion conveyed in a single experience of care hits home, lands hard and can silence a room. I've also noticed how well this information can be retained to remind us later to pay attention to the important things.

It's why, for me, the soft stuff is never soft.

> *A gentleman was critically ill in one of our hospitals – he had let the team caring for him know that he wanted to die at home, but they knew his condition meant that he would never survive the journey. Rather than just accept this as a sad fact, as he approached the end of life staff decided to act swiftly, holding the gentleman's wishes in mind.*
>
> *Quietly, without fuss, they closed the curtains of all neighbouring wards that overlooked a small contained courtyard. They didn't seek permission from senior leaders, or do a risk assessment, but they ensured privacy before moving the gentleman outside. Twenty minutes later he didn't die in hospital, he died in the garden, aware of the summer breeze on his skin and with his wife in his arms.*

Uncovering poor care

Leading the roll out of a patient experience programme is joyful and energising work when the feedback you have to share is extremely positive and enables staff to feel proud of what they do every day. However it is by its very nature a bumpy ride, because when you uncover poor practice as a leader you also have to ask yourself why it is happening and what can be done to support the staff to do a better job?

Within six months of real-time measurement I uncovered extremely poor practice on one ward in a small community hospital. The ward had no previous indications of poor performance with regards to safety; the level of complaints for the ward wasn't unusually high. In short there was a dark corner of our organisation that was completely off the radar.

Our first visit to the ward enabled us to speak to a group of predominantly older people who appeared to be fearful about speaking up and identifying those staff who were rough, cold and indifferent to their needs.

My emotional reaction on reviewing their initial feedback was naturally very strong; it was extremely hard to read the patients' comments and reconcile that it was our care that they were describing. I was upset and chose to return to the ward that evening and speak in confidence to relatives to gather further information about the extent of the problem. Information that I knew needed to be escalated immediately.

Years later, I still recognise the importance of the organisational response. Three members of staff were identified but nobody was dismissed in a knee jerk reaction. The Medical Business Unit immediately freed up time, showing an appropriate level of concern and an urgency to act. After receiving the feedback on a Tuesday, staff had been released for an away day by the Friday. There was a genuine desire to understand more about the staff experience, to recognise burn out and to listen to the barriers that existed to dignified care. It was also important to explore the climate of care that had prevented both patients and staff from raising concerns at an earlier stage.

Sunshine is the best disinfectant, so they say; owning this failure of compassion and talking openly about it, often, and right across our organisation and communities, was extremely important, but a very difficult thing to do.

I felt deeply for the gentle and kind geriatrician – clinical lead for the unit – who led the way in this regard. In every forum, he chose to tell the story without dismissing the reality of harm nor judging the staff responsible; at times his sadness and shame were palpable.

His genuine courage and leadership in the face of harm powerfully signalled to others that this had to be spoken about, it couldn't be rationalised or swept quickly away. In doing so he demonstrated that the organisation really did want to learn and improve, to do better by patients and their families, whilst also promoting a just culture for staff.

A comprehensive improvement programme was agreed and implemented. The team themselves defined new measures, standards and codes of conduct, including their own "always" and "never" events. They received funding for their immediate improvement priorities, which included dignity boxes for those patients who were unable to afford adequate nightwear, toiletries or personal care items of their own during their hospital stay. These dignity boxes found ways of promoting moments of connection, as nurses appreciated the time they had to sit quietly with patients as they gently applied hand cream.

The three members of staff were initially moved to other wards to learn from different teams. Importantly they then returned to the team with a shared responsibility to collectively make things better.

To avoid a quick fix, we focused instead on what it would take to evidence sustained change and improvement. We approached commissioners and requested that maintaining excellence in patient experience and dignity become part of an 18-month locally agreed CQUIN arrangement; critically it began with a very open and honest conversation.

I believe that this discovery of poor staff and patient experience in 2010 played an important part in the board finding more support and investment in the patient experience team.

I naturally welcomed the increased capacity for my team, but poor care had also taught me that I needed to broaden my measurement approach to find a voice for those who are seldom heard: the older people who are unable to participate in traditional surveys or experience interviews, due to the language and/or cognitive barriers that were in the way.

I established, in partnership with the third sector, an assessment framework to enable them, as recognised advocates of older people, to visit our wards and provide us with real-time feedback about the opportunities we took to promote dignified and respectful care, together with those we missed.

This work has not been without risk: it is certainly unusual for an acute organisation to routinely invite an external partner to observe their practice in this way. My hopes are that we will continue to provide an environment where we have the best chance of protecting some of our most vulnerable patients, and provoking questions where necessary about the way things have always been done.

When I originally designed our patient experience programme I consciously held patients in mind; what I didn't appreciate at the time was how much impact this way of working and improving would have on our staff. I've subsequently become very familiar with the evidence base and powerful association between staff experience and patient experience.

I remember one time when I was forced to defibrillate a patient as a matter of urgency in the early hours of the morning. I had to keep on reshocking the patient repeatedly. Defibrillation is not like how it's portrayed on the telly, on Casualty and the likes. This was brutal, utterly brutal.

I wanted to cry; I could feel the sting of tears in my eyes. But I had to keep goinog – this was urgent, and I was the one responsible for the outcome. But it was horrifically painful to see; to do. After it was over I ran to the store cupboard along the corridor, closed the door, and cried my eyes out for about a minute before collecting myself and moving on to the next patient.

Health care is emotionally challenging work. We deal with things which are difficult and unsettling and sometimes horrific. Sometimes one thing in particular can really strike a chord, and I think it is essential that we have the time and the space to process that emotion – to release tears, to grieve – if we are to be not only capable but also compassionate carers.

Staff experience precedes patient experience

The story above is shared anonymously on the Point of Care website and reveals an on-going challenge for NHS staff and organisations. Amidst the relentless demand and at times traumatic nature of delivering health care, how do we ensure our staff feel safe, stay emotionally engaged and equipped to continually give of themselves?

As early as 1959, Isabel Menzies-Lyth wrote about the need for nurses in organisations to emotionally protect themselves from the overwhelming nature of their job, particularly the need to keep human suffering at an objective distance in order to be able to successfully perform clinical tasks.

And yet admitting to compassion fatigue still feels taboo. I've heard more than one exec director of nursing express their dislike of the term, as if its very existence in health care was something to be ashamed of, and decidedly uncharacteristic of the nursing profession.

Within my role, I have taken every opportunity to use experience data to evidence the link between staff wellbeing and the care that patients receive. I've been lucky enough to work very closely with talented and committed colleagues in psychology, occupational health and human resources to raise awareness of these issues, and develop training resources on self-compassion and wellbeing.

Emotional stories like the one shared above are powerful. I feel motivated to learn when l hear these highly personal accounts of care and the feelings that underpin them. It's why experience based co-design has become my preferred improvement methodology.

Experienced based improvement

In 1999, when I was in a practice development role, I asked people using stroke services to describe how they felt at key stages of the stroke pathway; I colour-coded their responses into positive, negative and neutral comments and mapped these along our care pathway to help provide the team with a simple visual reminder of where we were meeting our patients expectations and where we needed to improve. I then asked staff to do exactly the same.

I later came to understand that this was my first clumsy attempt at emotion mapping and the beginning of a long standing commitment to co-production. I share this because I think it's a good reminder not to be afraid to trust my own emotional intelligence. Rather than wait to "find" the perfect QI tool, I should instead learn to trust my gut and follow my instincts to experiment.

Experience Based Co-design (EBCD) is an approach to improving care and services that has always instinctively appealed to me. EBCD emerged from the engineering industry and was adapted for health services in 2006, when Professor Paul Bates and Glen Robert argued that good design lay at the heart of quality health care.

It is a form of participatory action research that brings patients, staff and families together to share their experiences of receiving and providing care. It combines a person/user centred approach (EB) with a collaborative change process (CD), and as such has always felt entirely congruent with my values and the work I want to do.

The advantages of improving in a person-centred way are absolutely clear to me, but I wouldn't argue that EBCD is the only patient-focused approach. I recognise a commitment to understand the needs of the customer in many of the improvement methods, including LEAN's defining focus on delivering "value" as seen through the eyes of the customer.

For me, what separates EBCD from the other improvement methodologies is the co-production element. This approach doesn't just enquire about the patient experience, it commits to the active engagement of patients and families in the process of improving. This feels more meaningful and effective to me.

I adopt a fairly pragmatic stance when using EBCD. I've learnt to trust the group I'm working with at the time and adapt the application around their needs. I don't always follow all six stages (Figure 14.1) within the method, but I do honour and prioritise the joint meeting, the co-design, and the use of stories to inspire the heart.

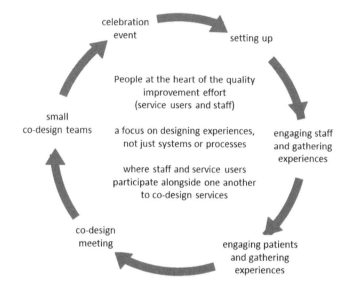

Figure 14.1

The time and space awarded in my role has enabled me to innovate and create novel approaches to quality improvement. The reality of messy application in clinical practice, and 25 years of NHS experience, has brought a freedom too which prevents me from being a slave to the textbook.

Maintaining the source of kindness for others: steps in self care

Understanding and promoting self-care has featured heavily in many improvement workshops that I have run for patients, families and staff. Practising what you preach can of course be a lot more difficult.

By December 2013, I was experiencing symptoms of burn out for myself.

I had been working very closely with another organisation that was in distress, and was travelling four hours a day, two to three times a week, to support the roll out of their patient experience programme.

Whilst working on the wards, it was easy for me to chuck myself in, heart and soul. As an extrovert I get my energy from people and relationships. I also have a strong need to be needed, particularly by those in pain and distress.

It was natural for me to feel acutely aware of the sadness I encountered in frustrated and powerless staff. At times I worried about emotional contagion, and whether just being around these strong emotions contributed to me feeling lonely, isolated and sad myself.

That year, I arrived in Ireland for the Christmas holidays and I felt disconnected and disorganised. I'd failed to provide my son's school and the dogs' kennels with adequate notice of our departure, my international presents to family were late and unwrapped, my UK cards remained unwritten.

For the first time ever I'd left our empty house undressed for Christmas, normally part of a joyful weekend and special tradition I share with my youngest son. I hadn't managed to fit in my usual drive round the village to check in with friends, and had sent regretful apologies for the team party for the second year in a row.

The realisation that I wasn't particularly concerned about the major surgery I was facing on 3rd January, because at least it would provide me with some rest, was perhaps the biggest indicator that I was seriously out of sorts.

I have come to recognise that by immersing myself in the concerns and needs of others, I can sometimes find a perfect distraction from the truth of what's happening in my own life. During these times I am able to silence my own needs or numb them with the heroics of important work.

In my fierce and frequent determination to "be strong" I can often deny myself the same rights of rest, play and happiness that I would want to fiercely protect for others.

For a long time I've seen my sensitivity as a weakness. I'd be emotionally moved by something and then feel embarrassed by my tears, or the fact that the colleagues beside me weren't reacting in a similar way. Internally, I hear a judgement that credibility lies with measured objectivity and emotional restraint that is inherent in professional behaviour.

And yet I believe that as human beings we are hardwired to connect intimately with others, and to naturally feel empathy when we witness pain, sadness, joy or distress. Open-hearted compassion inspires me to practise a deeply human approach to providing care to patients that I believe keeps me strong and resilient.

I discussed this with a trusted colleague and friend who likened my sensitivity to that of a sea sponge, sopping wet and therefore able to soak up all the emotions in the room, in contrast to other "drier" colleagues. She suggested that, at times, I may need to modify the holes in my sponge if I am to leave critical capacity to care for myself, and find the energy to play with those that I care about at home.

Over the last two years in particular I've recognised that my wellbeing, resilience and ability to sustain my own effectiveness as a leader is dependent on making some important personal changes. I've altered my role and committed to making my final decade in the NHS a far more playful one.

As I consider the exercises and actions that I could practise regularly in an effort to be kinder to myself, I question whether these needs aren't equally true for the teams that I work with and the organisations that employ us.

I have identified a number of provocative questions that I feel are important if we are to remain deeply close to the meaningfulness of our work without being overwhelmed by it.

- What would it mean for organisations, patients, staff, regulators, and commissioners if we sought first to understand the complexity in the system and then worked together, eyes wide open, to help improvement happen, as we are, where we are, without resorting to language of failure and shame?
- What if teams were given hope about the difference they could make, and given the means to work with patients and families and understand that we're all in this together?
- Would inspection still be necessary if timeout sessions provided teams with the skills to consciously pay attention to what was really happening on the unit/ward, in the moment, as it happened?
- What if, together, without blame, we felt able to take organisational responsibility for errors of the past and really learn from them?
- What if random acts of kindness, however small, became the way we got through our day and were regularly celebrated throughout our organisations?
- What if the new staff we chose to work with us understood, and had kindness and compassion stories of their own to tell?

The time is now

There is, in my view, something peculiar about the health care that, despite our core purpose as a "caring for people" business, we fail in so many ways to be customer focused. I genuinely don't understand why authentic patient engagement is still viewed as relatively novel when for almost every other industry the end user is the starting point of improvement and innovation.

I'm reminded that this isn't always about resources, but about attitude. An example includes a very small and humble garage in a rural part of Germany which used a simple and cheap technique to identify new and returning customers: a small sticker that the pump attendants would subtly place in the petrol cap whilst filling up with petrol. If a customer arrived without a sticker they treated the person as a new customer and went out of their way to encourage them to return. If someone arrived for petrol with their trademark sticker still visible, they welcomed the person back and thanked them for their loyalty.

By contrast, the NHS has people returning to them all the time and yet we don't retain information or share this well for the benefit of patients; we apply derogatory terms like frequent flyers to people with complex and multiple needs. In many ways the actions of seriously overwhelmed staff and services signal a message that they would prefer it if their customers would go away.

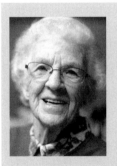

I am a patient – I am not a number above a bed or on a waiting list. I am not defined by my disease, my symptoms or health care condition.

I am the subject matter expert on how I experience my care and whether it meets my needs.

As I move through the service that you provide, I see things that you don't see and hear things that you don't hear.

I will hold creative solutions that you haven't thought of yet; work with me to deliver care that matters.

I heard a story recently that made me smile, about a nurse who was working on a ward when she noticed some water on the floor. Recognising a potential safety hazard, she called for a member of the domestic team to come and clear it up. The domestic arrived and looked at the floor; she was disappointed to see what she felt was a very minor spillage. Feeling frustrated that she'd been called away from other duties to do something that the nurse could quite easily have taken responsibility for herself, she shared her views, bluntly. A heated debate ensued, all conducted in front of a patient who lay in bed invisible and bemused.

Eventually, tired of the squabble, the patient rose to his feet, poured the content of his water jug on the floor and said "Tell me, is it big enough for one of you to do something about now?"

I share this story to reflect the frustration I sometimes feel about the rigidity of QI theory and methodology, and the scant regard that, I feel, is given to patients as active partners in improvement.

I sometimes wonder how big our problems have to get before we embrace a very different way of working.

I also share this story as a moment of personal reflection. As I read over my words, I can't escape my inherent judgment of staff. I notice how easily I've fallen into a trap of blaming their inaction, rather than blaming the system that was causing them to feel potentially pressurised and overwhelmed by the number of tasks that they had to do that day. On a much larger scale, I am frequently saddened by the extent of blame and shame in our regulatory system, for example, and how staff are currently having to shoulder blame for failings in the system that are entirely outside their sphere of influence. I am conscious of how harmful this is to both their psychological safety and creating the right conditions that will allow staff to speak up and own improvement. If what I want is to witness more compassion and less judgment in our system, then I need to be mindful of my own responsibilities within that, and the importance of consistently modelling the behaviours that I wish to see.

This causes me to reflect on the immense task of bringing about rapid improvements in NHS care and patient safety at a time of unprecedented workload pressures and increasing financial constraint – a myopic focus on efficiency and simply doing more with less is not what we need.

Chronic workforce shortages and high levels of work-related stress present barriers to high-quality and compassionate care that are, for me, every bit as great as the fiscal challenge.

If we are to avoid the huge decline in the scope and ambition of the services we provide, then it's my view that we need to work with patients, service users, families and the public in a very different way, to allow new and creative solutions to emerge.

It is also my belief that we will do this best by paying attention to the humanity of our interactions and the importance of a thread of kindness that weaves between these: the kindness we want our patients to always receive, the kindness we want our staff to naturally feel because they too feel cared for themselves, and the kindness we want our organisations and communities to embody and authentically promote. As Atul Gawande once put it so beautifully:

> *The notion that human caring, the effort to do better for people, might make a difference, can seem hopelessly naive. But it just isn't...*

(2008, p. 10)

I've reached a lovely stage in my career when I am able to choose the work I wish to prioritise and the people I wish to partner with in order to bring energy to the task. It is a freedom that has allowed me to affirm my own commitment to my organisation and to a wider effort to help the NHS to improve from within.

In a recent discussion with my Chief Executive about priorities for the year ahead, I've decided to return to basics. With a new role as Chief Experience Officer, I will have responsibility for improving staff experience as well as patient experience. This is a new post for our organisation, and the first of its kind in the NHS. I'm excited by the prospect of building appreciative systems that allow us to reliably and relentlessly acknowledge everything our teams do every day to support our amazing NHS. This will involve revisiting fundamental principles, measuring staff experience in real time, and taking the time to first understand what matters most to staff *before* we try and improve it. I feel confident about the support and commitment that I can rely on from my organisation. I also feel hopeful about what lies ahead. My focus is to create a legacy which means that a therapist, working late on our stroke units in the future, won't need to ask her colleagues "What is this organisation doing about person-centred care?" because she will already know.

Closing Reflections

Our contributors have told their stories. Perhaps the stories say what needs to be said without further interpretation.

Certainly, we do not intend to try to draw out some generalised truths about how you should lead quality improvement, nor devise some leadership competency framework which defines how superhuman you must be to have a chance in this arena. Although formulas, frameworks and models can sometimes help us make sense of what is going on, there is never going to be a single step-by-step approach which will meet the complexity of what you, as leader, are trying to do to meet the challenges we outlined in Chapter 1.

It does seem, however, too abrupt to end this book without at least some reflections on what we have been working with for a number of years, and what you have had some flavour of in the stories. These are our reflections, and you will have yours – perhaps together we can construct some abiding thoughts which will be helpful to you in your role.

Being aware of your own power – finding it, acknowledging it, working with it

There are many types of power. Often when we think about power in organisations, we think about positional power – the power conferred upon us by our place in the hierarchy. If I am the Medical Director and you a junior doctor, I have the power to instruct you to undertake a task; and if we abide by social conventions and the contract of our employment, you are pretty much obliged to carry it out.

The funny thing is, this kind of power seems from our stories to be one of the least effective in leading and sustaining quality improvement. Whenever one of our contributors starts down that path of thinking, "I will make this happen – I will tell them to follow this method", warning bells should start to ring. Often there is initial compliance, but compliance is not change, nor is it improvement.

A different kind of power, "soft power", is that which arises when human beings collaborate and decide together that they want to make a difference. The leader's job becomes how to help people to come together and to decide that this is what they want to do. Here the leader's power can be enormously helpful, offering support, sponsorship, protection, and encouragement.

If Fellows struggle with power, it seems that they often fall into one of two camps, and these are both recognisable in our stories. The first is an over-reliance on the positional power, and a tendency to advocate rather than inquire, to assume that by saying "make it so", that their job is done. The second is to not recognise their power, and to give it away. Although we contend that leaders cannot "make it happen", leaders' actions and role-modelling are still powerful. For some who have found themselves in a position of authority, this is sometimes hard to come to terms with, and they frequently underestimate the impact they have on their local context.

The stories suggest that there is a delicate course to be steered where power is concerned. Denying its existence or using it like a battering ram to force compliance appear to be flawed strategies in leading improvement. Instead, a more balanced use of power to support and encourage, and to invite collaboration, seems to be most effective.

Starting with small gestures

The grand plan, the big idea, the transformational change, the launch, the high profile internal communications, the sweeping change – all sound seductive and exciting. How else will we make things different around here? But equally effective, perhaps in the long term much *more* effective, are those initiatives which start small, with the chance conversation, with the discussion about "what do we want?", with the invitation to just begin something. Starting small allows contribution and shaping by those who are going to do the work, and therefore reduces concerns. It is liberating for those making the small move, because anxieties are reduced, and it doesn't matter if it doesn't work. You can learn from it, and make other small moves elsewhere, feeling your way forward, taking advantage of leaps in progress and contributions from others.

Moving, acting, having courage

It's perhaps an obvious thing to point out, but if you want things to change, action is required. Closely linked with the small gestures point above, your actions can start small but nonetheless they often require courage. It is understandable that when faced with what appears to be opposition, hostility, corporate inertia, or just the overwhelming complexity of it all, it can be tempting to just sit back and wait until next week, or next month, or next year, before beginning.

Sometimes on the GenerationQ programme we use the phrase "being ten percent braver". Our encouragement to the Fellows is not to become paralysed by the overwhelming circumstances they face, but to find the courage to just begin. Without that action, nothing changes; once that first step is taken, everything is possible.

Creating the conditions where improvement can happen

In the stories, a further theme is that people need the right conditions to be in place for them to flourish and to bring their creativity and energy to the improvement. They need to feel they are valued, that their contribution counts, that they have the freedom to act, and that they will be supported when they do. An essential job for the leader is to create these conditions. An obvious metaphor seems to be one of preparing the soil for the plants to flourish – the leader must do some work, tilling and digging, removing obstacles, feeding and encouraging. In the early stages, the seedlings need almost constant attention and reassurance, but once they are through this initial period, they become robust and self-sufficient, and need only occasional re-visiting to check on progress.

Offering enough structure – the toolkit and beyond

The title of this book, *Beyond the Toolkit*, conveys the high value we place on the toolkit of improvement methods. Improvement methods provide a number of powerful things for those involved in improving quality. Firstly, they provide a way of beginning, a structure which enables people to channel their enthusiasm and energy into purposeful ways of acting together. Without structure, we may not know where to start, which part of the process we should change first. We may not be clear about what it is exactly that we are trying to improve, or what is the scope of our improvement activity. We may try many different alterations to a process or a pathway, without knowing whether what we have done has been an improvement. Having a structure can be very helpful in reducing anxiety over what to do and how to prioritise.

Secondly, improvement methods provide a language for people to use in improvement. Having a shared improvement vocabulary can be invaluable in bringing people together and in helping them to effectively shape their joint endeavour.

Thirdly, improvement methods give a broader possibility for similar changes to be adopted more widely. We say possibility, because effective spread of improvement is still a complicated area which has seen mixed results in different contexts. But if we are all singing from the same hymn sheet, we have a chance of moving forward together across a broader landscape.

And, as explained in Chapter 3, we believe that in addition to the technical skills, a leader of quality improvement needs to have contextual, relational and personal leadership skills too.

A reflection on our contributors

In writing the stories which form the heart of this book, our contributors have undertaken an act of leadership which should not go unrecognised. The book has taken many months to write, and inevitably that has been a period of uncertainty for them. Nonetheless they have offered their stories freely and courageously, without knowing how the whole volume will look, and without knowing how their particular story will land with the reader. This is an act of courage, which they have generously made, because they are passionate about health and social care and want to share their experiences with you, and for you, in the hope that this will inspire, or reassure, or help you in some way. We are always humbled by the work that they do, and this act has just added to the respect we have for them.

Finally, we hope that this collection of stories has been useful to you, the reader. If this book has made you nod in agreement, or helped you to begin some improvement, or just reassured you that you are on the right track, then it has done what we intended. If it has given you inspiration and belief about improving health and social care and your role in doing so, we are delighted. There is much more on the subject of hope in the companion book to this one, *Hope Behind the Headlines – local leaders shifting local cultures*. We cannot deny the complexity and difficulties of the landscape in which you are trying to make lasting improvements. But if more health and social care leaders felt inspired and hopeful, who knows what might be possible?

Unpacking our mental models about organisations and leadership

As organisations are complex phenomena, researchers and thinkers have often drawn on metaphors to understand the nature of them more deeply. Metaphors help convey complicated concepts by referring to the properties of something which is familiar to us, in order to help understand something else which is not. So, when Shakespeare wrote in *As You Like It*, "All the world's a stage, and all the men and women merely players. They have their exits and their entrances", he was using the metaphor of a stage (something we can easily understand) to convey something about the nature of a much more complicated concept (the world). But herein also lie some of the difficulties with metaphors. Firstly, they only work for some aspects of the comparison. Although the world may in some ways be like a stage, with us always playing a role and never really seeing each other as we are, in other ways the world is not like a stage. We don't literally have lines to learn or speak. We are not consciously aware of performing before an audience. A further problem with metaphors is that we can easily fall into the trap of forgetting that we are using a cognitive, linguistic device to understand a complicated concept.

Machine thinking – the dominant metaphor

So what metaphors are used to describe organisations? The most dominant metaphor is seeing organisations as types of machine. Just as an engineer will design a machine by defining the different interdependent parts, so organisations can be conceived as a network of parts with interdependent functional departments. Within each functional department each job is precisely defined, all rationally organised, planned in an orderly fashion, and mapped onto a hierarchical organisation chart. People are in effect seen as cogs in the machine. Policies and procedures specify what each part of the organisation should do, when and how, very much as you would with a machine. There are inputs and outputs, and value is added by producing something or altering things that pass through it. Looking at organisations through this metaphor, it is unsurprising that standardisation, replicability and efficiency are the goals.

This metaphor, perhaps because it has been around so long, has become the dominant way of thinking about organisations in health care, as well as western organisations more generally. Without being consciously aware of this metaphor, the thinking and language it evokes have seeped into the way people talk. For instance, how many times have you heard people talk about engendering change by "pulling the levers", or that something has to be "well-oiled" if it is to "run" well?

The underlying comfort offered by the machine metaphor is one of control: the assumption is that machines can be made to do what we want. To effect change, all that is required is for output to be amended by fairly simple parameter alterations. The process can be changed, as can inputs or raw materials, and there is an assumption that people, like machine parts or cogs, will do what is required.

Looking at organisations through the machine metaphor has implications for how we understand leadership. The leadership required is highly directive, as the task of leadership is to ensure that people do as they are told and reliably perform their function. This in turn makes planning, measurement and control important. There is an assumption that control of the organisation as a whole is possible and lies with those at the top. Control can be through governance procedures, reporting lines and management by objectives. Deficiencies are identified and understood through diagnosis, problem solving and linear cause and effect, so that the organisation can be steered towards desired and predictable outcomes – again from the top. Indeed, the more a leader knows about a situation the more tightly he can manage what happens and the better the outcome achieved, hence the value placed on technical expertise.

These ideas have morphed into the idea of the leader as hero, which still has significant currency and influence today. One researcher, Gronn (2002), calls it "a belief in the power of one". There has been no shortage of leaders willing to publish self-aggrandising memoirs that fuel such a view. Management gurus too have furthered the notion of the heroic leader by introducing the idea of the transformational leader: someone who shares a powerful vision, is charismatic and inspires others to follow them. This view of leaders casts them as saviours when they turn around an organisation's fortunes, and utter failures when they don't. However, "by honing so relentlessly upon an individual, [this view of] leadership tends to blind us to the complex, social nature of particularly large organizations" writes Grey (2002).

Indeed, whenever we use a metaphor, it focuses our attention on some aspects of a phenomenon to the exclusion of others. This limits what we see and means we can unwittingly ignore other aspects. In envisaging the organisation as a closed entity, this metaphor diverts our attention away from the organisation's context and the environment, which is often the source of much unpredictability and things we can't control. People and how they respond, interact and relate to one another are a further source of unpredictability when leading change, yet the machine metaphor gives people a very limited role, seeing them as neither sources of creative energy and innovation nor of resistance.

> *Although the origins of this way of thinking about organisations can be found in the early part of the last century, the implications ricochet and reverberate within organisations today and lie at the heart of why many change efforts fail.*

> (Wiggins and Hunter 2016, p. 10)

Complexity thinking – an alternative metaphor

An alternative perspective on organisational life is based on the complexity sciences. This is illustrated by the "butterfly effect" – the idea that tiny initial changes can lead to substantially different outcomes elsewhere in the world. In the case of the butterfly, a small flap of the wings produces a storm on the other side of the globe. There may well be cause and effect, but it is not linear, and not possible to trace. Complex systems such as the weather and quantum physics are also impossible to control or predict, and this kind of thinking has been applied to other complex systems, in this case, organisations.

A writer we recommend on the GenerationQ programme is Ralph Stacey (2012). He was inspired by the complexity sciences, and the idea that organisations may be complex and unpredictable like weather systems. He sees organisations as operating in what complexity thinkers call "bounded instability". It is possible to predict certain large-scale and short-term things about organisational life, just as we know that, weather-wise, it is unlikely to snow in the Sahara. Our predictions have a certain boundary outside of which events are extremely unlikely but longer term predictions or more detailed ones are impossible in the weather and in organisations. This concept alone can be alarming for leaders as they begin to consider the implications of not being able to "control" their organisation in any predictable way, because organising is actually an ongoing process made up of many interactions between human beings.

If organisations are viewed through the perspective of complexity thinking and cannot be controlled or their trajectory predicted, what does this mean for leaders trying to improve things? Does this mean that they can do nothing? Will the organisation, like the weather, do its own thing, in spite of the leader?

Working with the idea of complexity

A common initial reaction to being introduced to these concepts is to believe that leaders have no influence over the direction our organisation will take. As one Fellow said, having attended her first GenerationQ workshop:

> At the forum I felt disturbed by the idea of complexity thinking. It seemed to beg the question "why bother?" If everything is ultimately chaotic, if diversity and difference are key to progress and whatever happens comes about by unregulated and uncontrolled processes, if the organisation only exists within the personal interactions of individuals, what is the role of the leader and what is the purpose of leadership? What had I been doing with my life so far?

However, the metaphor of the weather does not entirely fit all aspects of organisations. This is because leaders are very much a part of what goes on. Leaders may not be in control in any linear cause and effect sense, but are still powerful participants, whose words and actions have an effect.

Direction and meaning in organisational life emerge not from the actions of one individual but from the interactions *between* people. This is not a one-off event, but is a constantly repeated process of what Stacey calls "gesture and response".

To illustrate this with an example :

I decide I would like to launch a quality improvement initiative, and so I begin to talk to people about this idea. I speak to my boss, who responds enthusiastically to what I suggest, and I notice his response towards me (i.e.

his gesture), then when I speak to a peer next my gesture to her is shaped by my previous encounter with my boss. She reacts with unexpected enthusiasm and I feel very much heartened and thus her response also changes what I say and do. Meanwhile my boss has mentioned my idea to someone else and the dance of gesture and response goes on. This dance could at any stage come to a grinding halt, or could blossom into something new and exciting, or fall into familiar patterns. One of our Fellows writes:

> I have learnt about complexity thinking and the importance of paying attention to our gestures and how others respond. By paying attention to this level of interpersonal interaction I have found a shift in my relationships which has led to a richer quality of dialogue and quite rapid changes.

The point is, my gestures count. They may not get me exactly what I want or expected. They may have no effect, or more effect that I intended, but they still count.

Working with this concept is much more familiar to us all than it sounds. We are all constantly involved in this dance, and it is one that we are used to. We all know the feeling when our ideas are changed and shifted by those we work with, ignored by some, adopted by others, stolen by a few. And we also know how *we* change as we interact with others: that initial concept quickly seems to become naïve or too slow as others' responses to our gestures begin to shape the concept in our minds. However, so often we act as though this is not how things work, and instead return to our plans and our simplistic thinking, and then are surprised and disappointed when things don't turn out how we expected.

Why how we see and talk about organising is important

So why is this view of the organisational world important? Is it just an intellectual exercise or an examination of common ways of thinking, or does it have practical implications for how you do your job and how you lead ?

As a leader, how you think shapes what you do in very real and practical ways. If you believe that your organisation is a machine, then you will act in ways which are consistent with this. You will see control as vitally important and view yourself as *the* person in the driving seat. Anything and everything which feeds into this image of you as a leader driving and controlling the organisation will be part of your everyday actions. You will pay attention to, and be exceptionally sensitive to, plans, and the more detailed the better.

You will want data, hard data, to increase your level of control and certainty. Everything must have a process, so that you can enforce adherence to that process. When people have new ideas, you will want a detailed presentation of those ideas, and will be concerned with measuring progress. Targets are a vital part of your arsenal, because they enable you to instantly see if the machine is functioning efficiently, or if any of the parts need replacing.

Success, from the machine perspective, is a question of better enforcing adherence to all the structures and processes you have put in place. Difference and diversity are, at best, unhelpful, distracting you from moving as a single unit towards the goals which you, as leader, have chosen.

This may seem at first like an extreme interpretation of the behaviours originating from a machine view of organisations. However, you will perhaps recognise these behaviours as part of the standard approach to leading in health care with plan, review, control and grip, being the dominant words which have currency in this world.

What then if you entertained the view of organisations through the perspective of complexity thinking? What difference would this make to how you enacted your leadership? The first thing to say here is that this approach forces you away from a prescription, or a "how-to" guide of leadership. As soon as you lay out a simple "do this, in order to get this" approach you have fallen back into a view which tries to force cause and effect linear relationships, rather than embracing the complexity of organisational life. Leadership turns out to be much more improvisational and flexible than any formula of success could encapsulate.

Complexity thinking offers a more nuanced and sophisticated view of how leadership works. If you adopt this view, you will not expect things or people to simply comply with your wishes or your expressed intentions. Instead you will be deeply interested in how people respond to your gestures, paying attention to what they say and what they don't say. You will be prepared to be changed, trying to keep the balance between your intention and the meaning that is emerging in your interactions. Doing this requires you paying attention to what is going on for yourself and for others. It requires, therefore, using your third eye.

In all likelihood, you will start to see patterns in the organisation ways of doing things which are familiar and repetitive. Sometimes you will see these patterns as unhelpful and want to disturb them, recognising that this may cause anxiety in others, but also knowing that this is where new ideas and creativity can arise.

You will attempt to pay close attention in the present moment. With this new view of organising you know that different ways of doing things and opportunities for improvement can arise in every moment, and that if you look out for them, and amplify and encourage them, they sometimes become the starting point for something exciting. When something different is happening in a conversation, you will have the courage to see where it goes, rather than shutting it down and re-emphasising control. You will embrace informal processes and conversations as well as formal processes, and spend time engaging with people, whether that be one-on-one, or in small and large groups, and facilitating high-quality conversations. You will still recognise the value of plans and data, recognising that some structure is really useful. However, you will be mindful of the fact that a plan never happens exactly the way you thought it would and that data only tells a very small part of the story.

Above all, taking complexity thinking seriously means recognising that organising is a social endeavour that happens between human beings. Your ability to work well with others will be a key factor in shifting patterns, in helping find energy and motivation, and in getting the momentum needed for quality improvement. And sometimes things will not go as planned. This is not an indicator of poor leadership, or a bad plan. As the stories show, this is simply what happens when human beings come together in the collective endeavour known as organising. Perhaps the biggest shift in our Fellows is that they find they can accept the messiness of complexity thinking, they are able to helpfully reframe any setbacks as an opportunity for learning.

Relational dynamics

In this appendix, we offer a short precis of four relational theories that are mentioned in the contributors' stories. For more in-depth coverage of these, and further topics such as navigating politics, using power and designing effective meetings, the interested reader is referred to: *Relational Change: The art and practice of changing organizations,* Wiggins, L. and Hunter, H., 1st ed. Bloomsbury, 2016.

Here we consider the following:
1. Transactional Analysis
2. The drama triangle and the winner's triangle
3. Push and pull / directive and facilitative change
4. Dialogue

1. Transactional Analysis

This theory, Transactional Analysis, often abbreviated to TA, is a wonderfully rich theory that embraces ideas from psychoanalysis, behavioural psychology and humanistic philosophy. "TA is a way of inquiring into what goes on between people and inside people in order to help them make changes. The transactional aspect is exactly what it says: a two way communication, and exchange, a transaction", writes Charlotte Sills (2011). A transaction can take place internally when we talk to ourselves, or between two people, and it does not have to be verbal. It might be a raised eyebrow or a sharp intake of breath at someone's comment. In this respect it is similar to Stacey's ideas of gesture and response explored in Chapter 3. The analysis involves looking at these interactions in ways which help us to understand them and structure them so that we can make helpful changes.

TA locates the source of our responses in what the originator of the theory, Eric Berne, called three ego states: Adult, Parent and Child. These three ego states are "coherent systems of thought and feeling manifested by corresponding patterns of behaviour" (1967). According to the theory, we are in an Adult ego state when we are thinking, feeling and behaving in the moment and are therefore really "present", alive to the here and now and what is going on. There is no interference from the past. There are two unconscious reservoirs of past experience, known in TA as the Child ego state and the Parent ego state. These are generalisations of past experiences which become habitual and stylised ways of responding to similar stimuli. What makes a pattern become fixed is the level of stress or emotion that was aroused in the original experience. Other people's behaviour, or emotional situations, can trigger us to respond from the Child or Parent ego state, rather than the Adult. When this happens we are responding in the same way we did in the past.

In the Parent ego state we have unconsciously taken inside ourselves messages and experiences from others, generally our own parents, carers and teachers. So we have "introjected" key messages that gradually, through reinforcement, become part of our script, our way of understanding and experiencing the world. There are two aspects of the Parent ego state – the Critical Parent and the Nurturing Parent. Signs of being in the ego state of Critical Parent would be telling other people what to do; using the words "should" and "ought" a great deal; a tendency to use quite extreme adverbs such as "you *always* mess up"; "you *never* do as you are told". The Nurturing Parent shows concern for the other person's feelings and wellbeing; has a gentle tone of voice; tries to make things better for the other person, even if it fosters dependency.

When we are in the Child ego state we are reliving ways we behaved as a child. Here again there are two aspects: the Free Child and the Adaptive Child. In the ego state of Free Child, feelings of joy, fear, sorrow, distress are expressed in a very uninhibited way. This ego state allows spontaneity and creativity, but may not see, or be aware of, risks. The ego state of Adaptive Child means that behaviours are adaptions to others' gestures. When in the Adaptive Child ego state, an individual may be *rebellious,* dig their heels in, question and challenge the authority of another, or express anger when sadness would be more appropriate. Alternatively, when in the Adaptive Child ego state, an individual may be *compliant*, cowering with head down as they ask something from someone else, trying to guess what might please or placate the other. Their voice tone in this ego state is likely to be whingey or placatory and they express fear where anger would be more appropriate.

The relevance of this to leading improvement, and change in general, is that many of the behaviours or gestures we encounter in others, or indeed may experience ourselves, are quite likely to derive from the Parent or Child ego states, given that change evokes strong emotions. If someone speaks to us from their Parent ego state it can easily trigger us to respond from our Child ego state. Conversely if someone is in a Child ego state we can find ourselves almost automatically responding from our Parent ego state.

Transactions which "complement" each other are those where there is a match. Gestures and behaviour from an Adult ego state invite behaviour from a complementary Adult ego state in the other person. However, thoughts and subsequent behaviours from either Parent or Child ego states invite behaviour from the other which reinforces the Parent to Child or Child to Parent transaction.

Thus, if someone you meet adopts a parental, critical tone, and tells you how things should be, you may well feel the temptation to respond in a way which is from the Child ego state, agreeing meekly or feeling childishly rebellious. Similarly, if someone comes to you in a Child ego state with a whole set of worries and issues, they may be inviting you to take a parental nurturing position and relieve them of all their concerns.

Obviously, if we are aware of this, we may decide not to follow this pattern of Parent-Child complementary transactions and instead react from a more Adult state: being clear about our boundaries and our responsibilities, accepting what is ours, and declining what is not. This form of refusal to play is called a Crossed Transaction in TA.

If you are aware of your own responses, by using your third eye you can sense which ego state others are coming from, and can consciously choose to respond from a different ego state. Indeed the very act of noticing and choosing is a mark of being in the Adult Ego state. For genuine dialogue, being in Adult is important, and if you can stay in Adult you can often help the other person to get back in touch with their own Adult ego state too. For those times when you want innovation and creativity, the ideal ego state would be that of Free Child, for at least part of the time.

2. The drama triangle and the winner's triangle

Developed by Karpman in 1968 (referenced 2011), the drama triangle (see Figure Appendix 2.1 below) describes three characteristic positions that people may take up in interactions with others: victim, rescuer and perse-cutor. In each position people replay ineffective patterns of thoughts and behaviour, getting hooked by other people's responses and in turn hooking them, so that everyone becomes locked in a vicious dance. The drama triangle can also occur in the conversation we have with ourselves in our heads. We will each have a predisposition to one position but can unconsciously get hooked into any of them, depending on other people's responses. We, and they, can also move around the positions. Getting out of the pattern requires one or more people being able to spot the pattern and notice what is happening, which equates to being in an Adult ego state. The different positions can be described in the following way:

> **Victim**. *In the position of victim people tend to feel fearful, singled out and self- pitying. The type of phrases characteristic of someone occupying this position are "It's all too much for me", "Why does this always happen to me?", "I've got so much going on for me you can't expect me to...", "He's always picking on me", "It's the fault of the system". In TA terms, when in this position, an individual is in the Child ego state.*

> **Persecutor**. *In the position of persecutor people tend to feel threatened, pressured and right. The type of phrases characteristic here are "You are always making excuses". "We'd be OK if it weren't for...", "It doesn't matter what you feel, just get on with it". In TA terms, in this position, the person is in the ego state of Critical Parent.*

> **Rescuer**. *In the position of rescuer people tend to feel capable, overburdened and righteous. The phrases here are "I'm carrying everyone", "I'll sort it out", "They can't manage so I'll do it", "Don't worry about me". In TA terms, this position is that of Nurturing Parent.*

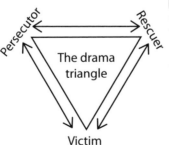

It's all your fault!
- Critical, blaming, controlling, sense of superiority
- Act in own interests
- Part of their goal is to punish
- Often Critical Parent

Poor you! Let me help.
- Concern for the victim
- Take over the thinking and problem solving
- Do more than their share
- Do things they don't want to do
- Often Nurturing Parent

Persecutor · Rescuer · The drama triangle · Victim

Poor Me!
- Powerless, helpless, stuck
- Act as if they don't have the resources to solve their problem

Figure Appendix 2.1

Choy (1990) created a reframe of the drama triangle which he called the winner's triangle (see Figure Appendix 2.2) in which all the positions are Adult so that the victim becomes the creator, the rescuer becomes the coach and the persecutor becomes the challenger.

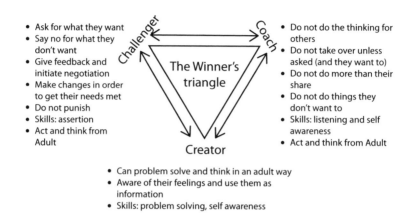

- Ask for what they want
- Say no for what they don't want
- Give feedback and initiate negotiation
- Make changes in order to get their needs met
- Do not punish
- Skills: assertion
- Act and think from Adult

Challenger

The Winner's triangle

Coach

- Do not do the thinking for others
- Do not take over unless asked (and they want to)
- Do not do more than their share
- Do not do things they don't want to
- Skills: listening and self awareness
- Act and think from Adult

Creator

- Can problem solve and think in an adult way
- Aware of their feelings and use them as information
- Skills: problem solving, self awareness

Figure Appendix 2.2

3. Push and Pull; directive and facilitative change

Here we look at the sources of energy in relationships, depending on the type of intervention between individuals, or indeed a leader and a group of people. John Heron (2009), a pioneer in the field of participatory research methods, was fascinated by the impact of different ways of asking questions and commenting in one-on-one conversations. He developed a model which is a useful way to explore the different styles open to us when we interact with each other. He began his research looking at how GPs inter-acted with their patients, but later looked at interactions between people in numerous work settings. He differentiated between "push" and "pull" inter-vention styles. By intervention, he means ways of asking questions or making comments, indeed anything that could be called a move, or what Stacey[2], would call a gesture. "Push" gestures are more directive; "pull" more facilitative.

For many leaders, the behaviours that go with a directive approach to change are familiar, as they tend to fit with the dominant machine metaphor view of organisations, and the idea of the leader as someone who tells others what to do. However, to engage others in change and create the conditions for innovation, it is vital to develop and use the pull styles. The pull behaviours which are required in order to adopt a more facilitative approach sometimes need a little more attention and practice.

Pull interventions encourage others to open up, to share their thoughts and feelings and what they notice is going on, to become more aware of what they believe or know, to give more of themselves, to be engaged. Such interventions put others in the driving seat in terms of directing the content of a conversation or discussion. They are therefore particularly helpful when you are wanting to find out what others are noticing and experiencing. Being open, listening well and genuinely being curious are important here.

One of the Fellows described what he noticed – in retrospect – when he tried to introduce Lean:

> *I never stopped to think "Are my colleagues ready for this change?"*
> *Lean talks of Pull and Push systems [Womack and Jones, 2003]. Push*
> *systems require an excessive effort to propagate the process. However,*
> *Pull is where flow is effortless. I have realised that the phenomenon of*
> *Push and Pull were playing out in front of me, but not in the processes,*
> *rather in my relationships with colleagues. I had been pushing my*
> *ideas onto them – an incredibly energy sapping and inefficient way of*
> *fostering change and a good way of stimulating antibody production*
> *in those around me. This reminds me of the work of Heron [2009] who*
> *described both Push and Pull intervention styles. The similarity*
> *between Heron's work and Lean became real to me. I needed more Pull*
> *and less Push. The only difference is that Lean would say Push is*
> *always wrong and the perfect system is entirely based on Pull.*
> *However, I have learnt from this that Push is sometimes required. I*
> *had needed to initiate this change with Push to create awareness that*
> *things could be different, and then convert to Pull.*

4. Dialogue

Dialogue is a theory associated with Bill Isaacs (1999). He was interested in ways to ensure that conversations harnessed the collective intelligence of a group, by creating settings where people can safely and consciously reflect upon their differences through inquiry and listening to each other. By asking "pull" questions and then really listening to the responses, people begin to loosen the grip of certainty they might have been carrying. Isaacs introduces the important idea of suspending. By this he means letting go, for the moment, our beliefs and assumptions. Instead, in dialogue the encouragement is to attend to the present rather than reliving and re-seeing through our memories of old hurts, slights, beliefs and stereotypes. This then allows people to begin to see things from new perspectives, and then new ideas and understanding emerge in unexpected and fruitful ways. This shared inquiry becomes a way of thinking and reflecting together, and "from shared meaning, shared action arises".

When we are in debate or discussion we seek to win in some way through defending a position, often one which was been held unchanged throughout the conversation. In dialogue, we are ready to listen and be changed by what we experience with others.

This requires a skill which in theory most people think they have, but which in practice seems often severely lacking – that of listening. Hearing is not listening. Often in conversations with others we think we are listening, but actually we are just waiting for our partner to stop talking so that we can make our brilliant point. Really listening is not a passive act; it requires us to be fully present and to allow others in.

Personal drivers

As children, we create a narrative, or "life script", for ourselves about how we see our life which is based largely on the numerous encouragements, reprimands and cajoling we received from parents, care-givers and our early teachers. For example, I may hear the message from parents based on a few incidents about how clumsy I am, and this may stay with me for life – a belief that I am just "that sort of person" who will always be a little clumsy. Kahler and Capers (1974) found that these life scripts contain the need for approval, driven by beliefs that "if I am like this, then I will be acceptable". They identified five main "drivers" of behaviour:
- Please People
- Be Strong
- Be Perfect
- Hurry Up
- Try Hard

These social messages are probably all recognisable to you, but the likelihood is that some will have greater personal resonance than others because you were exposed to them more frequently, or perhaps some came with far greater rewards or sanctions attached. Being socially pleasant, striving to be our best, putting in effort – all of these things can be extremely beneficial in our lives. More problematic is when one or two tend to really dominate and begin to "drive" us in ways which can be unhelpful to ourselves and others. Thus, if I have a strong belief that I should Be Strong, I may be reluctant to ask for help, soldiering on as a hero and alienating everyone around who has tried to offer support. If I have a Please People driver I may go to great lengths to avoid conflict with others, even though an honest conversation might be genuinely needed.

In the stories, the Fellows often use the drivers to catch themselves in the heat of the moment, thinking "Is this just my Hurry Up driver at play? Do we actually need to slow down to get the best out of this situation?" or, "Am I just Trying Harder because that's part of my upbringing? Perhaps the answer is not simply more effort". Leaders have told us that the notion of personal drivers has helped them understand other people's emotions and explain occasional strong emotional reactions they experience. However, although our personal drivers can be helpful for us as adults to navigate our way in social situations, we often act them out automatically. In leading improvement, they can prompt us to respond in a default way, rather than pausing to think whether this is a helpful response right now or remember that each has a shadow side.

Be Perfect   If you have a Be Perfect driver you are the sort of person who believes things should be the very best they can be. You strive for high standards, and expect the same of others, and you pay attention to detail. You get annoyed when documents have typos or the percentages on a graph don't add up to 100. With this behavioural driver, it can be difficult to delegate, as it can be hard to trust others to do as good a job as you would do. People with a Be Perfect driver can sometimes be seen by others as intense and picky.

Be Strong   Those who have a Be Strong driver are able to stay calm under pressure and are the people you want around in a crisis, as they remain emotionally detached, are great at problem solving and are reliable. Many doctors have this driver. The shadow side is that people with this driver can find it hard to ask for help or to admit any difficulty. Such people can therefore seem very private, uncaring, non-communicative or withdrawn. Their greatest fear is that if they show their vulnerabilities they will be scorned or rejected by others. In terms of leading improvement, the default for those with this driver can be to try and solve all the issues themselves, but in doing so they risk alienating or excluding others who can and would like to be involved.

Hurry Up   Those with a Hurry Up driver love being busy and thrive when there is lots to do. They tend to be fast workers who respond well to short deadlines. The shadow side of this is that they will often delay starting something until it is urgent, and may then make mistakes if they are in too much of a hurry or have treble booked themselves – a fairly frequent behaviour in those with this driver. They find people who take a long time to get their words out rather annoying, and dislike silence or having nothing to do and too much time to think. Others can find such people frenetic, agitated and annoying when they make demands on colleagues to hurry up. They can also have the unfortunate habit of finishing people's sentences for them. The challenge for those leading improvement who have a Hurry Up driver is to slow down and recognise that others need time to think, to explore, to get up to speed with what is under discussion.

Try Hard   People with this behavioural driver tend to be enthusiastic and put a great deal of energy and effort into projects. They are particularly great to have at the beginning of projects as, along with this enthusiasm, they are often creative and have a broad outlook. The shadow side is that they can sometimes put in much effort without necessarily achieving a great deal, and can create mountains out of proverbial molehills, or easily get distracted. Their greatest fear is being told they haven't tried or are irresponsible. Others can see such people as sulky, rebellious, taking on more than they can handle. Leaders with a Try Hard driver benefit from having others around who can help them stop and evaluate whether the effort is productive.

Please People   Those with this driver like harmony. They are good team players who will try not to ruffle feathers unduly; they will be empathetic, helpful and encourage good relationships among others. However, this can mean that they are not always sufficiently assertive on their own account and can sometimes take on other people's issues. Being rejected, criticised or ignored are their greatest fears. Others can see such types as people who are unable to say "no", get overly involved emotionally, and help others in order to feel better about themselves. The challenge for leading improvement for people with this driver is to recognise and accept that when instituting changes it is impossible to please everyone. A level of disagreement is inevitable, and the important thing is to neither avoid tough conversations nor take them personally.

A self-assessment questionnaire to help you identify your dominant drivers is included below.

Personal Drivers questionnaire

Completing the questionnaire:

Study every section listed in the table below, carefully, reading through the five statements listed. From these five statements pick out the one which is the **most true** for you and give it a high mark (between 7 and 10) in the right-hand column. Then find the statement that is **least true** for you and give it a low mark (between 0 and 3). Then arrange the other three statements in between, giving each a mark which ranks them between your lowest and highest. Please ensure that one statement is given a mark of 5.

Scoring the first section may take a little while. Once you get going the others will not take as long. The whole questionnaire should take between 20 and 30 minutes to complete.

Section		Statement	Score (0-10)
1	a	Endurance is a valuable asset.	
	b	I like to see people doing their best to get things right.	
	c	Considering all the effort I put into things I should get more done.	
	d	I find myself doing too many things at the last minute.	
	e	On balance I adapt more to other people's wishes than they do to mine.	
2	a	Casualness and carelessness bother me.	
	b	It's keeping on doing things that interests me more than finishing with them.	
	c	When people are slow about saying something I want to interrupt or finish the sentence.	
	d	I have a fair amount of imagination when it comes to guessing what people need.	
	e	When someone gets emotional my reaction is often to make a joke of it or else be critical	
3	a	I don't mind things being hard. I can always find the energy.	
	b	I prefer to use just the minimum necessary time to get to a place.	

Section		Statement	Score (0-10)
	c	If someone doesn't like me I either try hard to get them to like me or I walk away.	
	d	It is rare for me to feel hurt.	
	e	If it's a question of doing something properly I'd rather do it myself.	
4	a	I get impatient with slow people	
	b	Normally I prefer to take people's wishes into account before deciding something.	
	c	I show a calm face even when my feelings are running high.	
	d	I don't make excuses for poor work.	
	e	There's something about coming to the end of a job that I don't like.	
5	a	I put a lot of effort into things.	
	b	Sometimes it is better to just do something and leave the discussion until later	
	c	I'm cautious about asking favours.	
	d	I don't let people look after me much.	
	e	I sometimes find it hard to stop myself correcting people.	
6	a	Sometimes I talk too quickly.	
	b	I'm uncomfortable when people are upset or displeased with me.	
	c	I dislike people making a fuss about things.	
	d	Things can always be improved on.	
	e	I don't believe in the "easy" way.	
7	a	I think I do a lot to be considerate towards others.	
	b	I usually manage to cope even when I feel I've had more than enough.	
	c	I prefer doing things really well even if it takes longer.	
	d	I tend to start things and then gradually lose energy or interest.	
	e	I want to get a whole lot of things finished, then I run out of time.	

Section		Statement	Score (0-10)
8	a	I'm not what you would call soft.	
	b	I prefer to do things right first time, rather than have to re-do them.	
	c	I sometimes repeat myself because I'm not sure I've been understood.	
	d	My energy is often at its highest when I have a lot of things to do.	
	e	It's quite hard to say no when someone really wants something.	
9	a	I like to use words correctly.	
	b	I like exploring a variety of alternatives before getting started.	
	c	It's quite like me to be already thinking of the next thing before I have finished the first.	
	d	When I'm sure someone likes me I am more at ease.	
	e	I can put up with a great deal without anyone realising it.	
10	a	People who just want to finish something tend to irritate me.	
	b	I prefer to just plunge into something rather than have to plan.	
	c	If a person doesn't know what I want I'd rather not have to ask directly.	
	d	Other people start whining and complaining before I do.	
	e	I prefer to correct myself rather than have other people correct me.	
11	a	If I had 20% more time I could relax more.	
	b	I often smile and nod when people talk to me.	
	c	When people get excited I can stay very cool and rational.	
	d	I can do something well and still be critical of myself.	
	e	There are so many things to take into account it can be hard to get to the end of something.	

Section		Statement	Score (0-10)
12	a	I have a good intuitive sense if someone likes me or not.	
	b	I think duty and reason pay off better than emotion in the long run.	
	c	I tend to see quickly how something could be improved on.	
	d	Some people have a habit of over-simplifying things.	
	e	Sometimes the more there is to do, the more I get done.	

Table Appendix 3.1: Adapted from de Haan and Kasozi (2014)

When you have finished scoring all the sections, transfer the marks onto the scoring sheet (Table Appendix 3.2) below, listing each mark you have given it against the appropriate letter (a, b, c, and so on) and add them up to give you a total for each of the five drivers.

Personal Drivers' questionnaire: scoring chart

Question number	Item number	Your score	Item number	Your score	Item number	Your score	Item number	Your score	Item number	Your score
1	a		b		c		d		e	
2	e		a		b		c		d	
3	d		e		a		b		c	
4	c		d		e		a		b	
5	d		e		a		b		c	
6	c		d		e		a		b	
7	b		c		d		e		a	
8	a		b		c		d		e	
9	e		a		b		c		d	
10	d		e		a		b		c	
11	c		d		e		a		b	
12	b		c		d		e		a	
Total	Be Strong		Be Perfect		Try Hard		Hurry Up		Please People	

Table Appendix 3.2: Adapted from de Haan and Kasozi (2014)

References

Preface

Deming, W. (1982) *Out of the Crisis*. Cambridge Mass: Massachusetts Institute of Technology, Center for Advanced Educational Services.

Godfrey, M. (2012) *Team Coaching – Sheffield Microsystem Coaching Academy*. Available from : http://www.sheffieldmca.org.uk/UserFiles/File/Coaching_one_page_book_V5_Final.pdf

Introduction
Section 1 Framing
Chapter 1: The Challenges of Leading Improvement

Berwick, D. (2002) A User's Manual for the IOM's 'Quality Chasm' Report. *Health Affairs*, 21(3), 80-90

Berwick, D. (2013) *A Promise to Learn – a commitment to act: Improving the safety of patients in England'* published by Department of Health and Social Care. Available at https://www.gov.uk/government/uploads/system/uploads/attachment_data/file/226703/Berwick_Report.pdf. Accessed March 2018

Binney, G., Wilke, G., and Williams, C. (2012) *Living Leadership: a practical guide for ordinary heroes*. 3rd ed. Harlow: Pearson Education Limited

Brown, M. (1998) The Invisible Advantage. *The Ashridge Journal*. Nov 1998, p. 20

Charlesworth, A., Thorlby R., Roberts, A. and Gershlick, B. (2017) *Election Briefing: NHS and social care funding. Three unavoidable challenges*. London: The Health Foundation

Fillingham, D., Jones, B. and Pereira, P. (2016) *The Challenge and Potential of Whole System Flow*. London: The Health Foundation. Available at http://www.health.org.uk/sites/health/files/ChallengeAndPotentialOfWholeSystemFlow.pdf . Accessed March 2018

Gregory, S., Dixon, A., and Ham, C. (2012) *Health Policy under the Coalition Government: a mid-term assessment*. Retrieved from https://www.kingsfund.org.uk

Lafond, S., Charlesworth, A. and Roberts, A. (2016) *A Perfect Storm: an impossible climate for NHS providers' finances? An analysis of NHS finances and factors associated with financial performance*. London: The Health Foundation

McCandless, K. (2008) *Safely Taking Risks: Complexity and Patient Safety*. Retrieved from https://www.med.uottawa.ca

Rittel, H. and Webber, M. (1973) Dilemmas in a General Theory of Planning. *Policy Sciences 4, 155-169*. Available at https://doi.org/10.1007/BF01405730. Accessed March 2018

Stacey, R. (1996) *Strategic Management and Organisational Dynamics*. London: Pitman Publishing

Wiggins, L. and Hunter, H. (2016) *Relational Change: The art and practice of changing organizations*. London: Bloomsbury Publishing plc.

Stiehm, J. and Townsend, N. (2002) *The U.S. Army War College: military education in a democracy*. Philadelphia: Temple University Press

Chapter 2: The Toolkit

Bate, P. and Robert, G. (2006) Experience-Based Design: From redesigning the system around the patient to co-designing services with the patient. *Quality & Safety in Health Care*, 15(5), 307–310. Available at http://doi.org/10.1136/qshc.2005.016527. Accessed March 2018

Goldratt, E. and Cox, J. (2004) *The Goal: A process of ongoing improvement*. Aldershot: Gower Publishing

Knight, A. (2014) *Pride and Joy*. Aldbury: Never Say I Know

Langley, G., Moen, R., Nolan, K., Nolan, T., Norman, C. and Provost, L. (2009) *The Improvement Guide: A Practical Approach to Enhancing Organizational Performance* (2nd edition). San Francisco: Jossey-Bass Publishers. Available at http://www.ihi.org/resources/Pages/HowtoImprove/default.aspx

OECD (2017), *Tackling Wasteful Spending in Health*. Paris: OECD Publishing

Scoville, R., Little, K., Rakover, J., Luther, K and Mate, K. (2016) *Sustaining Improvement*. IHI White Paper. Cambridge, MA: Institute for Healthcare Improvement (Available at ihi.org)

Springham, N. and Robert, G. (2015) Experience based co-design reduces formal complaints on an acute mental health ward. *BMJ Open Quality*, 2015; 4:u209153.w3970. doi: 10.1136/bmjquality.u209153.w3970

Womack, P. and Jones, D. (2003) *Lean Thinking.* London: Simon & Schuster UK Ltd.

Chapter 3: Beyond the Toolkit

Berne, E. (1967) *Games People Play.* London: Penguin Random House

Brown, B. (2012) *Daring Greatly.* 1st ed. London: Penguin Random House

Brown, B. (2010) *The Power of Vulnerability.* [on line] TED. Available at: https://www.ted.com/talks/brene_brown_on_vulnerability. Accessed 27.02.2018

Buchanan, D. and Boddy, D. (1992) *The Expertise of the Change Agent: Public Performance and Backstage Activity.* London: Prentice Hall

Clance, P. and Imes, S. (1978) The Imposter Phenomenon in High Achieving Women: dynamics and therapeutic interventions. *Psychotherapy: Theory, Research and Practice*, 15 (3) pp.241–247

Heifetz, R. (2002) *Leadership on the Line: Staying alive through the dangers of leading.* Boston, MA: Harvard Business School Press

Heron, J. (2009) *Helping the Client: a creative practical guide.* 5th ed. London: Sage

Isaacs, W. (1999) *Dialogue and the Art of Thinking Together.* New York: Doubleday

Jepson, D. (2009) Leadership context: The importance of departments. *Leadership and Organization Development Journal* 30 (1): 36 – 52

Kahler, T. and Capers, H. (1974) 'The Miniscript'. *Transactional Analysis Journal*, 4, (1) 26 – 42

Kolb David A. (1984) *Experiential Learning: experience as the source of learning and development.* Englewood Cliffs, Prentice Hall :1984

Lapworth, P. and Sills, C. (2011) *An Introduction to Transactional Analysis.* London: Sage

Pedler, M., Burgoyne, J. and Boydell, T. (2004) *A Manager's Guide to Leadership.* McGraw-Hill Business

Shaw, P. (2002) *Changing Conversations in Organizations: a complexity approach to change.* London: Routledge

Watzlawick, P., Weakland, J. and Fisch, R. (1974), *Change: Principles of problem formation and problem resolution.* New York: W W Norton

Wiggins, L. and Hunter, H. (2016) *Relational Change: The art and practice of changing organizations.* London: Bloomsbury Publishing plc.

Section 2: Experimenting
Chapter 4: Shouting at a Flower Doesn't Make It Grow

Heifetz, R. and Linksy, M. (2002) *Leadership on the Line: Staying alive through the dangers of leading.* Boston, MA; Harvard Business School Press.

Isaacs, W. (1999) *Dialogue and the Art of Thinking Together.* New York: Doubleday

Lapworth, P. and Sills, C. (2011) *An Introduction to Transactional Analysis.* London: Sage

Solberg, L., Mosser, G. and McDonald, S. (1997) The three faces of Performance Measurement: Improvement, Accountability and Research. *Journal on Quality Improvement.* March 1997, Vol 23, No. 3

Chapter 5: Lessening the Roar

NHS Improvement (undated) *SAFER patient flow bundle.* Available from https://improvement.nhs.uk/resources/safer-patient-flow-bundle-implement/

Repenning, N. and Sterman, J. (2001) Nobody Ever Gets Credit for Fixing Problems that Never Happened: Creating and sustaining process improvement. *California Management Review*, Vol.43, No.4 Summer 2001. Available at http://web.mit.edu/nelsonr/www/Repenning=Sterman_CMR_su01_.pdf. Accessed April 2018

Chapter 6: Getting Out of the Way

Langley, G., Nolan, K., Nolan, T., Norman, C. and Provost, L. (2009) *The Improvement Guide.* California: Jossey-Bass Publishers, Inc.

Shaw, P. (2002) *Changing Conversations in Organizations: a complexity approach to change.* London: Routledge

Chapter 7: Moving through Treacle, Discovering Pearls

Stacey, R. (2012) *Tools and techniques of leadership and management : Meeting the challenge of complexity.* London: Routledge.

Section 3: Engaging
Chapter 8: Reframing and Seeing the World Differently

Karpman, S. (2011) Fairy Tales and Script Drama Analysis. *Group Facilitation*, (11), 49

Lapworth, P. and Sills, C. (2011) *An Introduction to Transactional Analysis*. London: Sage

Chapter 9: Riding the Waves

Binney, G., Wilke, G., and Williams, C. (2012) *Living Leadership: a practical guide for ordinary heroes*. 3rd ed. Harlow: Pearson Education Limited

Isaacs, W. (1999) *Dialogue and the Art of Thinking Together*. New York: Doubleday

Stacey, R. (2012) Tools and Techniques of Leadership and Management: Meeting the Challenge of Complexity

Streatfield, P. (2001) *The Paradox of Control in Organisations*. London: Routledge

Wiggins, L. and Hunter, H. (2016) *Relational Change: The art and practice of changing organizations*. London: Bloomsbury Publishing plc.

Chapter 10: Leaning Out and Letting Go

Brown, B. (2012) *Daring greatly: How the courage to be vulnerable transforms the way we live, love, parent, and lead*. New York: Gotham Books

Heron, J. (2009) *Helping the Client: A creative practical guide*. 5th ed. London: Sage

Lapworth, P. and Sills, C. (2011) *An Introduction to Transactional Analysis*. London: Sage

Law, D. and Jacob, J. (2015) *Goals and goal based outcomes (GBOs): Some useful information*. 3rd ed. London: CAMHS Press

Sandberg, S. (2015) *Lean In: Women, Work and the Will to Lead*. London: WH Allen

Williamson, M. (1992) *Return to Love: A reflection on the principles of a course in miracles*. London: HarperCollins

Chapter 11: Joining the Pack

Brown, B. (2010) The Power of Vulnerability. [on line] TED. Available at: https://www.ted.com/talks/brene_brown_on_vulnerability. Accessed 27.02.2018

Goffee, R. and Jones, G. (2005) Why should anyone be led by you? *Harvard Business Review, 1*, p64

McCandless, K. (2008) *Safely Taking Risks: Complexity and Patient Safety.* Retrieved from https://www.med.uottawa.ca

Shaw, P. (2002) *Changing Conversations in Organizations: a complexity approach to change.* London: Routledge

Section 3: Committing
Chapter 12: Improvement Is the Work

Block, P. (2007) *Civic Engagement and the Restoration of Community: Changing the nature of the conversation.* Retrieved from http://www.asmallgroup.net/

Chapter 13: Daisy

Chapter 14: The Thread of Kindness

Berwick, D. (2009) What "Patient-Centered" Should Mean: Confessions of an extremist. *Health Affairs* , 28, 560–562.

Gawande, A. (2008) *Better: A Surgeon's Notes on Performance.* London: Profile Books

Closing Reflections
Appendix 1: Unpacking our mental models

Grey, C. (2002) The Fetish of Change. *Tamara: Journal of Critical Post Modern Organization Science* 2, (2) : 1 – 19

Gronn, P. (2002) Distributed Leadership as a Unit of Analysis. *Leadership Quarterly.* 13 (4) : 423 – 5

Stacey, R. (2012) *Tools and Techniques of Leadership and Management: meeting the challenge of complexity.* London: Routledge

Wiggins, L. and Hunter, H. (2016) *Relational Change: The art and practice of changing organizations.* London: Bloomsbury Publishing plc.

Appendix 2: Relational dynamics

Berne, E. (1967) *Games People Play*. London: Penguin Random House

Choy, A. (1990) The Winner's Triangle. *Transactional Analysis Journal*, 20 (1); 40

Heron, J. (2009) *Helping the Client: a creative practical guide*. 5th ed. London: Sage

Isaacs, W. (1999) *Dialogue and the Art of Thinking Together*. New York: Doubleday

Karpman, S. (2011) Fairy Tales and Script Drama Analysis. *Group Facilitation*, (11), 49

Lapworth, P. and Sills, C. (2011) *An Introduction to Transactional Analysis*. London: Sage

Womack, P. and Jones, D. (2003) *Lean Thinking*. London: Simon & Schuster UK Ltd.

Appendix 3: Personal drivers

de Haan, E. and Kasozi, A., (2014*) The Leadership Shadow: How to recognize, and avoid derailment, hubris and overdrive*. London: Kogan Page London

Kahler, T. and Capers, H. (1974) 'The Miniscript'. *Transactional Analysis Journal*, 4, (1) 26 – 42

About the Authors

The authors co-lead GenerationQ, a Master's programme in Leading for Quality Improvement for senior leaders in health, social care and health charities. The programme is sponsored by the Health Foundation and designed and delivered at Ashridge Executive Education, Hult Business School.

Brian Marshall is Academic Director and Discipline Lead for OD and Change at Ashridge Executive Education, Hult International Business School. Former roles include Strategy Director for Unipart and head of OD at the UK Civil Service. Brian has a first degree in English literature from London University, and a Master's degree in Organisational Change from Ashridge.

Janet Smallwood has also been involved with GenerationQ since the outset of the programme and has more than 20 years' experience as an OD consultant and leadership developer. She holds Masters Degrees in Natural Sciences and Chemical Engineering from Cambridge and the Ashridge Masters in Organization Consulting.

Liz Wiggins is Associate Professor of Change and Leadership at Ashridge Executive Education, Hult International Business School and has over twenty-five years' experience of working with leaders in the US, Europe and Asia. She worked as a leader herself at Unilever and Smythe Dorward Lambert and has two Masters degrees and a PhD in Organizational Psychology from Birkbeck College, University of London.

Contributors. The stories are written by senior leaders who participated in GenerationQ and they provide rarely heard, personal, "warts and all", accounts of what it is like to lead in practice, making moves to improve things for the better in their workplaces.